Healthy Longevity
without
Dementia

Healthy Longevity without Dementia

Dr. Richard Ng, B.S., D.O.

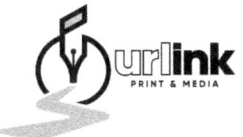

Healthy Longevity without Dementia

Copyright © 2024 by Dr. Richard Ng, B.S., D.O.. All rights reserved.

No part of this publication may be reproduced, stored in a retrieval system or transmitted in any way by any means, electronic, mechanical, photocopy, recording or otherwise without the prior permission of the author except as provided by USA copyright law.

The opinions expressed by the author are not necessarily those of URLink Print and Media.

1603 Capitol Ave., Suite 310 Cheyenne, Wyoming USA 82001
1-888-980-6523 | admin@urlinkpublishing.com

URLink Print and Media is committed to excellence in the publishing industry.

Book design copyright © 2024 by URLink Print and Media. All rights reserved.

Published in the United States of America

Library of Congress Control Number: 2024907262
ISBN 978-1-68486-749-3 (Paperback)
ISBN 978-1-68486-752-3 (Digital)

12.03.24

Mission Statements

1. To inform the public, the families, caregivers, healthcare providers and friends for better understanding of Alzheimer's disease and related dementias, to dispel any of the myths about dementia, and to encourage and bolster awareness of the mitigating and aggravating factors in the development of the dementia.

2. To give sincere supports to the loving, grieving and steadfast caregivers on their long, grueling journey with their silently-suffering loved ones.

3. To help individuals with dementia to have some quality of life and dignity with as much as independence and inter-dependence in their struggles.

4. To support continuing medical research in collaboration with beneficial cultural input, positive social changes, NGO involvements, and non-partisan governmental policies so that we can defeat dementia in 20 years, within my life time at my current age of 70.

5. To promote and achieve healthy longevity, and to reduce social burden and human sufferings of dementia.

Contents

1: Introduction ix
2: The Five Blue Zones 1
3: Lifestyle Changes for Healthy Longevity 8
4: Nutrition and longevity, the dietary approach to a healthy, long lifespan: 33
5: Dementias 70
6: Treatable and reversible dementia 87
7: Post-operative Delirium and Dementia 107
8: Signs and Symptoms of Dementia in General 111
9: Factors that increase the risk of dementia 117
10: Memory and Dementia 148
11: Inflammation and dementia 154
12: Dementia's impact on the caregivers: 160
13: Epilogue 167

Introduction

With the advances in our medical knowledge and technology, people are living longer, but that does not necessarily mean that we are living healthier. Living more years in poor health is actually not what most, if not all, the older people want; this causes not only a lot of financial stresses, grief and sadness for both the patients and caregivers, but also carries a stupendous burden for the society.

As of the year 2020, the numbers of adults aged over 30 made up half the total global population, marking the start of an increasingly aging world. The world's older population, the geriatric group, continues to grow at an unprecedented rate. About 9% of the people worldwide are aged 65 and over. This percentage is projected to jump to nearly 17 percent of the world's population by 2050 (1.6 billion approximately). In the U.S., the 65- and over- population is projected to almost double from the current 54 million by the year 2050. This undoubtedly will increase the number of Americans needing long-term care services.

Aging is a multi-faceted process in which bodily structures and functions undergo a negative deviation either gradually or quickly from the optimum --- growing old. The time of life when age-related physical and physiological changes appear depends on a variety of factors:

- Genetics
- Diet
- Culture
- Activity levels
- Environmental exposures
- Mental health and well-being

As you can see, there is very little, if any, you can change in your heredity; the other factors are within your control to modify and change for betterment, meaning you can do something about it.

Aging, in general, is the process of becoming older, with biological changes over time that lead to deterioration and eventually death. There are several theories about aging: the aging-clock theory, the genetic theory, the immunological theory, and the free-radical theory. The free-radical theory is the most commonly accepted theory at the present time; it is based on the fact that on-going bio-chemical reactions of the cells in the body produce free radicals which are harmful to the body under oxidative stress.

Everyone knows their chronological age with their birthdays, unless they have and are suffering from memory issues. We are used to measure age chronologically, counting the number of candles on your last birthday cake. However, do you know your biological age (or health age)? Chances are, like most of the people, you probably don't. Biological age has a lot to do with what is going on inside your body, and the goal is to bring this age down. In actuality, biological age is essentially the same as physiological age. There are different methods of calculating or estimating your biological age, applying and using different parameters. To make yourself biologically younger, it is not one-size-fits-all; it is quite individualized when it comes to lowering your biological age.

The Biological Age calculator starts with your actual age:

Based on your body weight,

- Add 2 years, if you are obese
- Add 1 year, if you are overweight
- Minus 1 year, if you are underweight
- Minus 2 years, if your BMI is normal and physically fit

Based on your physical activity levels,

- Add 2 years, if you do 150 minutes of aerobic exercise weekly
- Add 1 year, if you try to walk as much as you can

- Minus 2 years, if you do no exercise and walk very little

Based on your levels of mental stimulation,

- Minus 2 years, if you are learning a new language, or a new music instrument
- Minus 1 year, if you enjoy reading or playing video games
- Add 2 years, if you just sit down and watch TV all the time

Based on your diet,

- Minus 2 years, with a balanced diet of 75-80 percent fruit and vegetables
- Add 1 year, diet is not plant-based, with fried and junk foods most of the time
- Add 2 years, living on fast food and convenience meals with sweets

Based on your job,

- Minus 2 years, if you are active and do not have a sedentary job
- Add 2 years, if your job is sedentary, sitting about eight hours a day
- No change essentially if you are able to move around and to get up and down every hour at your job

Based on smoking history,

- Minus 2 years, if you are non-smoker, and not around smokers
- No change, if you don't smoke anymore despite smoking history
- Add 2 years, at least, if you smoke regularly

Based on your sleeping habits,

- Minus 2 years, if you have at least 7 hours of quality sleep most of the nights, waking up and feeling refreshed
- Add 2 years, if you sleep less than six hours a night
- Add 2 years at least, if you struggle with sleep all the time

Based on alcohol consumption,

- Minus 1-2 years, if you have one or two glasses of red wine occasionally
- Minus 1 years, if you do not use alcohol
- Add 2 years, if you drink everyday including wine, beer and liquor

Based on your stress levels,

- Add 2 years, if you feel stressed all the time and find it overwhelming, with irritability and moodiness
- Minus 1 year, if you feel under short-term stress sometimes but able to perform your daily activities and enjoy being with family and friends

Biological age is a better health indicator than the numbers of years you have lived. No two people age the same way and rate. Biological age, in reality, is a more accurate measure of health-span---the number 0f years lived in good health. Some people are ' rapid agers ', experiencing a faster rate of functional deterioration relative to their chronological age. With the rapid growth of the world's elderly population, finding out ways to assess and measure biological age and how to maintain or delay its advance is not only critically important for individual health, but also for social, political and economic health for our society.

Biological age is multifaceted, and is influenced by many factors including genetics, microbiome composition, environment you live, lifestyle, stress levels, diet and exercise. Our genes probably account for about 20% to 30% of biological age. Researchers have identified genes that play a role in resilience and protection from stress, repairing DNA, protecting cells from free radicals and regulating fat levels. However, currently there is no effective test to measure biological age. There are some promising molecular markers that may serve as biological age fingerprints. One of the promising markers is epigenetics---chemical modification of DNA that control gene function, for example, DNA can get marked by methyl groups in a pattern that changes with age and could potentially act as a marker for aging. Another marker of biological age is the build-up of dysfunctional cells called senescent or zombie cells. These dying cells become senescent because they are so damaged that they cannot divide anymore, releasing toxic molecules that cause low-grade inflammation.

The American Heart Association coined the ' the essential 8 of life ', describing and recommending eight ways to slow down biological aging. As follows:

- Eat better – here you can have some healthy choices such as the Mediterranean diet, or follow your own meals with at least 80% plant based (fruits and vegetables).
- Move more – Being more active with regular exercise.
- Stop smoking – to avoid toxic substances and powerful free radicals.
- Get quality sleep, 6 to 8 hours a day.
- Watch and manage your body weight.
- Watch and control your cholesterol.
- Watch and manage your blood sugar – diabetes is notorious to cause damage to the heart, eyes, kidneys and nerves.
- Watch and manage your blood pressure (medications and/or diet).

Research has demonstrated that Biological age may be slowed significantly when people adopted the eight behaviors recommended by the American Heart Association.

The word " longevity " is sometimes used as a synonym for " life expectancy ". To be precise, the term " longevity " usually refers to especially long-living members of a population, whereas " life expectancy " is defined statistically as the average number of years remaining at a given age. Longevity has been the desire of humanity for thousands of years, and the topic for the scientific researchers, writers of science fictions and utopian novels. Many societies are aging fast, but their governments are ill-prepared. Indeed, it is a ticking time bomb!

The Five Blue Zones

Around the world, certain groups of people enjoy exceptionally long lives. The Pacific Islanders of Okinawa, Japan, have an average life expectancy of more than 81 years, compared to 78 in the U.S., and a world-wide average of 67. Here in the U,S., members of the Seventh Day Adventists, who typically are vegetarians, outlive their American counterparts by 4 to 7 years on average.

Residents of the San Blas Island off the coast of Panama very rarely suffer from hypertensive cardiovascular disease and enjoy a longer lifespan than the mainlanders. Indeed, researchers have found that their rate of cardiovascular disease is only 9 per 100,000 people, compared to 83 per 100,000 among the Panamanians on the mainland. More and more evidence suggest that diet is one of the important contributing factors to longevity and healthy aging.

Knight Templars' secret of longevity might lie in their unique diet, according to researchers. Their diets usually included lots of fruits, vegetables, legumes and fish, and drinking moderate amount of wine with aloe pulp. Their diets historically enabled the Knight Templars to live much longer compared to the people of the Middle Ages, whose life expectancy averaged 26 to 40 years.

Let us look at the five " blue zones " of the world where centenarians are common:

Okinawa, Japan --- a gregarious, closely-knit community with considerable social support through all of life's ups and downs. They value and maintain strong social ties, thus, reducing mental stressors and reinforcing shared healthy behaviors. It is unquestionably accepted by researchers and conclusively supported by many social studies that isolation and loneliness lead to shorter lifespan and premature death.

Japan, as a country, has the highest number of people per capita over the age of 100 than anywhere else in the world. Admittedly, there may be some genetic differences at play, but more importantly, there are also diet and lifestyle practices that lead to longer lifespan with fewer of the age-related chronic illnesses such as cardiovascular disease, type-2 diabetes mellitus, and Alzheimer's disease. Here are some of the habits that are rooted in the Japanese culture:

- Japanese diet is filled with many nutritious plant foods including seaweed. These marine plants are packed with minerals, such as iodine, copper and iron along with antioxidants, clean protein, fiber and beneficial omega-3 fats.
- A Japanese person in Japan eats about 70 pounds of seafood annually, compared to a typical American who consumes about 16 pounds of seafood a year.
- Japanese drink a lot of green tea, which is rich in polyphenol antioxidants. The green tea promotes gut health, where majority of the immune cells and neuro-chemicals are produced.
- Eating and enjoying the food with mindfulness is practiced by Japanese; they usually stop at eating when they are almost full, the 80% rule.
- Forest bathing is a form of nature therapy practiced and enjoyed by Japanese. Studies have shown that when compared to being in a city setting, being in a forest setting (or being outdoors) is associated with lower blood pressure, lower levels of stress hormone, cortisol, and an increase in para-sympathetic nervous system activity, which promotes the feeling of calmness.

Loma Linda, California USA --- this blue zone is a haven for the Seventh-day Adventist Church, a protestant denomination. Their emphasis and shared principle of community and adherence

to the Sabbath --- a day of rest, reflection and recharging --- help the resident-Adventists of Loma Linda live at least 10 years longer than their fellow Americans. It is noteworthy that many of them avoid meat, and a typical Seventh Day Adventist diet includes:

- Fruits – bananas, apples, grapes, berries, peaches, pineapple and mango
- Vegetables – dark leafy greens, broccoli, bell peppers, sweet potatoes, carrots, union and parsnips
- Nuts and seeds – almonds, cashews, walnuts, Brazil nuts, sunflower seeds, sesame seeds, chia seeds and flax seeds
- Legumes – beans, lentils, peanuts and peas
- Grains – quinoa, rice, amaranth, barley and oats
- Plant-based protein – tofu, tempeh, edamame and seitan
- Eggs – occasional
- Dairy – usually low fat

Sardinia, Italy --- a predominantly plant-based diet, regular daily activity and familial closeness have given this Blue Zone the highest concentration of male centenarians in the world. Most of the men are sheep herders, who usually walk at least five miles a day. Their plant-based diet is traditionally accented with lean meat. The classic Sardinian diet consist of whole- grain bread, bean, garden vegetables and fruits. They also eat pecorino cheese made from grass-fed sheep, whose cheese is rich in omega=3 fatty acids. It also does not hurt that the M26 marker, a genetic variant linked to longevity, has been passed down through generations in this secluded community.

Nicoya, Costa Rica --- the residents of this Blue Zone in Costa Rico tend to avoid processed foods and traditionally these Costa Ricans get the majority of their calories from beans, squash, corn and tropical fruits. Their plant-based nutrient-dense diet with plenty of outdoors activities promote strong, well-nourished bodies, along with devoted, guiding life purposes, many of them stay mentally-sharp and spiritually fulfilled to the age of 90 and beyond.

Dr. Richard Ng, B.S., D.O.

Ikaria, Greece --- this island of Ikaria has been around for a very long time. Historical records and archeological findings suggest that Ikaria has been inhabited since at least 7,000 B.C. Despite successive wars that caused great losses in human life, the people on this island live on. The older population of this island is mostly free of dementia and other chronic diseases. Their strong sense of self-respect and pride keeps the Ikarians invested and involved in this island community. Their strict adherence to the Mediterranean diet, which includes lots of fruits, vegetables, beans, whole grains, red wine with moderation in meats, keeps the islanders of Ikaria in Greece healthy, both physically and mentally with longevity. There are also other factors contributing to Ikarian' long healthy lives, which include their mountain lifestyle: the residents of this Blue Zone walk up and down hills maintaining muscle mass and dexterity for decades longer than most Americans. Research advises that it is important to work against gravity when exercising such as walking, performing squats and pushups.

Another interesting factor observed in the Ikarians is the inclusion of health-promoting herbs, like the popular rosemary, in their meals. Rosemary is high in polyphenols that help feed the good bacteria of your gut microbiome and are converted into life-extending compounds that help keep the entire body functioning optimally. If you do not like rosemary, you can try oregano, sage thyme, and basil with their high levels of polyphenols. Taking a nap in the middle of the day is common among the Ikarians; the naps help improve memory and mood and reduce stress. Last but not least, beyond what and how they eat, the centenarians of Ikaria make spending time with their loved ones and friends a priority; indeed, social interactions drive successful aging.

In the U.S., the richest Americans live at least 10 years longer on average than the poorest. Interestingly, while the income does decide your life expectancy to some extent, the locality in which you reside, your lifestyle you choose and the foods you eat also decide how long you will live.

Let us look at the life expectancy chart listed by the World Health Organization for the countries in the world. Japan is on the top of the list at 84.2 years, a combined figure of men and women; Switzerland has the second spot at 83.3 years, Spain at 83.1 and Australia at 82.9 years for the top four positions in the WHO 2021 list. Surprisingly, the U.S. ranked the 34th in that year with a life expectancy of 78.5 years, despite the fact that the U.S. is the wealthiest and most influential nation in the world.

In the Hungarian folk tale, a king is trying to find out what makes his son, the prince, so gloomy and depressed after staying abroad for a while. Is it love? Is he heart-broken? No, the prince has discovered a simple truth of life. " Alas!, your majesty ", answered the prince, " it is not love or marriage that makes me so gloomy; but the thought which haunts me day and night, that all men, even kings, must die. Never shall I be happy again until I have found a kingdom where death is unknown. And I have determined to give myself no rest till I have discovered the land of immortality".

One undeniable truth is 'none of us will live forever no matter what you do'. Another truth is ' aging is inevitable in life '. People, in general, do not think about aging as something that is treatable. Should aging be treated like a disease? If that is the case, it is a very, very common disease. The conventional and traditional medical approach has been to treat diseases as they appear. We have the unavoidable biological realities of aging, but recent medical and scientific advances have shown that the power to curtail some of its negative effects on our biology may be within reach and modifiable.

Researchers in geriatric science found that increasing ' healthy ' life expectancy by just 2.6 years could result in a $83 trillion value to the economy. This certainly would reduce the incidents of stroke, cardiovascular disease, cancer, dementia and frailty. Today, a person who turns 65 in the next few years will spend an average of $180,000 on long term care due to their disabilities, according to a recent report commissioned by the U.S. Department of Health and Human Services. Our focus should be preemptive and preventative, striving for health span to match lifespan. The impact of age-related diseases such as type-2 diabetes, cardiovascular disease, cancer, crippling arthritis and Alzheimer's disease will become more pronounced and challenging.

There is no doubt that modern medicine has increased life expectancy; in the past 100 years, the global life expectancy has more than doubled. This is because we eliminated most of the illnesses and health concerns that took people out in early life; problems like infectious diseases, difficulties at childbirth, infections, even accidents have been greatly reduced through the years. Unfortunately, many of those years from the increase of life expectancy are burdened by age-related chronic illnesses. It is important for us to understand the difference between health-span and lifespan: health-span is how many years we remain healthy and relatively free from those diseases or serious illnesses whereas lifespan is the total number of years we live. According to Worldwide Google searches, healthspan is lagging lifespan and the gap is growing. Age has been in the headlines in the years 2020 and 2021 during the COVID-19 pandemic, since older individuals, especially those with chronic diseases, are at a higher risk of becoming seriously or fatally ill from COVID-19.

Why do we care and talk about health-span? To improve and lengthen health-span to match lifespan is a topic relevant to all people with significant and huge social and economic consequences around the world. The treatments for improving our current health-span don't necessarily mean drugs; public education, social support, physical activities, a balanced diet, beneficial behaviors and habits without smoking and drinking alcohol, adequate sleep and stress reduction are important healthspan determinants. The leading causes of death in the U.S. include heart disease, lung cancer, stroke, Alzheimer's disease and Type-2 diabetes; they are more prevalent in people 65 and over. After all, what is a long lifespan worth if it does not include a long, matching healthspan? I dare to say that most of us, if not all, do not desire to stay alive after our health has completely deteriorated.

When you are asked about your age, it is referring to your chronological age. It is based on your date of birth and reflects how long you have been alive and how old you are. Chronological age keeps on going with the march of time. There is another kind of age, called biological age, and it is wise and definitely worth knowing about it. Biological age essentially refers to how quickly or slowly the intra-cellular components such as DNAs in your cells are aging or deteriorating within the organs. This is something you have the ability to control and change, unlike the inexorable march of time in chronological age. Biological age depends on a number of things such as nutrition, sleep, stress, environment (or your surroundings) and your lifestyle habits and choices. According to research with many studies, biological age is only 10 to 15 percent genetics, and you have the ability to modify it, to either tone down the 'bad' genes or tone up the 'good' genes.

Here is one very important and significant message: you can actually change your biological age to achieve a longer healthy lifespan! Biological age is not just an abstract concept or idea, but a quantifiable biometric that can be utilized in both preventive and curative medicine. There are blood tests that can be ordered and analyzed by medical professionals, with over 40 different biomarkers in order to assign a number to your biological age. If your biological age is high relative to your chronological age, it is not a death sentence; it is important to keep in mind that the test results are essentially a highly individualized personal health profile that can be used to target certain problem areas and ultimately turn back the 'clock'.

Lifestyle Changes for Healthy Longevity

Let us begin with things within your control that can add years to your life:

There have been many convincing studies with overwhelming research that show that remaining physically active, avoiding toxic habits, eating healthy foods, staying mentally agile and stimulated, having adequate sleep, and minimizing stress can dramatically influence your lifespan in a positive way. While you may not be able to control every eventuality, you can proactively influence your health in more ways than your parents and grandparents ever thought possible. It is difficult to convince people to focus and think of their health in a future tense. As long as I feel okay today, why worry? Ironically, this is just a big part of the problem in the first place. We must take more personal responsibility for our own health throughout our lifetimes, not just at the end of it.

- Walking --- It is the preferred method of exercise for the longest-lived people and centenarians on earth. Research shows that the average American walks about 4,700 steps or less a day while hunters-gatherers walk at least 15,800 steps every day. Our ancestors spent most of the day on their feet and work very hard to get food, dig and hunt; they managed to live close to the age of 70. Yet, the animal that is closest to us genetically, the chimpanzee, usually does not live more than 30 years. Compared to the humans, chimpanzees enjoy a fairly easy life, spending most of their day resting and sleeping on the treetops, picking fruit and eating seeds. You do not really need 10,000 steps a day to extend your life. University of Massachusetts Amherst researchers found that adults could benefit from less than that ' magic ' number in a comprehensive analysis of 15 different studies across four continents published in the Lancer in March 2022. They found that adults younger than 60 can benefit anywhere between 8,000 and 10,000 steps a day for improved longevity; for adults older than 60 years of age, longevity benefits stabilize around 6,000 to 8,000 steps a day with decreased risk of early death. The point is 10,000 steps is not the bare minimum for improved longevity; any extra movement helps and the more steps you can do, the better your health.

Older people in developed countries, in general, don't have to do any physical work. Today, we have a pension that guarantees that we do not have to work in old age, and this is a relatively new concept in human history. There seems to be very little discussion about appropriate physical activities for older people, even though we know how important it is to be active. Lamentably, many people after retirement do not want to get up too much from the recliner. We must remind ourselves to move more and lie down less because even small doses of physical activity can have a huge, positive impact on the rate at which we age.

Even light physical activity can change you at a molecular level; researchers have shown that exercise like regular walking 30 minutes, four to five days a week, by the older people can repair damage of aging at the molecular level in cells and tissues of the body. Regular walking, according to the studies, improve your chances of longevity because it can slow the aging process and reduce the risk of diseases like high blood pressure, type-2 diabetes, stroke, heart disease, cancer and neuro-degenerative disorders like Alzheimer's disease. Walking is relatively easy for most people, it does not require special shoes, it can be done anywhere essentially and it can be by those whose joints may be aggravated by running. Research has demonstrated that walking is as good for your heart as running.

One review of 14 studies about walking with data from at least 280,000 people, found that three hours of walking per week was associated with 11% reduced risk of death from all causes compared with those who did little or no activity. Thus, it seems clear that walking may extend your life!

Walking is a complex behavior and a very healthy function, but many of us in our modern digital world have taken it for granted or simply forget about it. Many people become sedentary in their lifestyles, night and day without realizing the serious consequences for their general health. The high cost of a sedentary lifestyle became more evident with a new global study showing that inactivity drives 1 in 14 deaths. These findings based on population data for 15 health outcomes across 168 countries, were published in March, 2021 in the British Journal of Sports Medicine.

Walking requires functional integration of a lot of sensory and motor interactions and experience; it activates the brain and the musculoskeletal system. One of the important components of walking is balancing. In order to maintain the body's balance unconsciously and effortlessly as it changes position and moves over somewhat uneven different terrain in a gravitational field, the brain needs and interacts with different information. It relies partly on a mechanism in the inner ears responsible for sensory orientation in three-dimensional space. If this function of inner ears fails, you cannot maintain equilibrium. Balancing is extremely crucial to minimize the risk of falling, especially in the geriatric group; many incidents of falling resulted in fractures such as the hips which would immobilize the elderly with significant health consequences.

As we age, we lose the ability to absorb sufficient calcium into the Body, and the bones become thinner, leading to osteoporosis. Osteoporosis is a common cause of fractures among the elderly, Hip fractures in particular. Statistically, hip fractures strike at least One out of three women and one out of six men. Walking Stimulates the body's assimilation of calcium and other nutrients.

A gradual exposure to the sunlight with walking could be a wonderful and natural way to increase your calcium absorption into the body and bones to minimize and/or prevent osteoporosis. Studies have shown that walking increases bone mass (bone density), not only in the legs, but also the arms.

Walking can help lowering the blood pressure because the movements open up the capillaries in the muscle tissues by reducing the resistance to blood flow in the arterial beds, causing the blood pressure to drop. It is universally agreed among researchers that a normal blood pressure helps to lower the risk of heart disease, stroke and Alzheimer's disease.

Walking burns glucose and decreases insulin resistance. As one gets older, insulin sensitivity decreases; walking can help improve insulin sensitivity and lower blood glucose levels. In other words, walking can improve management of diabetes and reduce its complications, promoting longevity. There is no magic formula for how many steps you should walk, despite the talks about a baseline of 10,000 steps a day. If you can do more, more power to you and you have everything to gain. It is important to get in the habit of walking every day if you are physically capable; just make it part of your daily routine --- something you do without even thinking about it.

- Optimism and positive attitude --- having a positive attitude with an optimistic approach will bring more happiness in your life, and happiness is strongly related to how long you will live. Maintaining a positive attitude is associated with longevity, according to a study of centenarians in 2012 in the Journal of Aging. Researchers from the Albert Einstein College of Medicine found a correlation between optimism and longer life span. A positive attitude toward life can be the difference between checking out early and being the last one at the party. This positive, beneficial trait can add up to 7.5 years to your lifespan according to many studies. A positive attitude or optimistic mindset allows you to see the world in a new light and clarity in situations even when things are going downhill. An optimist sees the glass half-full, while a pessimist sees the glass as half-empty. According to many studies published in Harvard Health, optimism helps people cope with disease and recover from surgery with positive impact on health and longevity. Having a positive attitude helps you build hope and believe in your abilities to strive harder. The attitude of the patients in their healing process is always one of their strengths as identified by their therapists. Recovering from a physical or mental trauma or abuse is faster if the patient maintains having a positive attitude and optimism throughout the therapy process.

Many studies have shown that people with heart problems who have a positive attitude are more likely to benefit from the impact. They also showed low statistics of hospitalization requirement and a better mortality rate. By eliminating the stress and anxiety from your life, positive attitude and optimism is the road to a vibrant, healthy and long life along with a sense of purpose for living. In other words, people who live longer tend to be optimistic and manage their stress well; they have remarkable resilience that mitigates age-related chronic diseases.

- Maintaining Oral Health can help improve overall general health. In a 2000 report of the Surgeon General named ' Oral Health in America ', it highlighted the national importance of oral health and its relationship to overall health. However, disparities, identified 20 years ago, have not been adequately addresses, and greater efforts are needed to tackle both the social and economic determinants that create these inequities and systemic biases.

The medical-dental divide is problematic because many people do not realize that oral health is so important. Poor oral health might contribute to various disease including endocarditis – an infection of the inner lining of the heart chambers or valves, typically occurs when bacteria or other germs from another part of the body, such as the mouth, spread through the blood stream and attach to certain areas of the heart.

Although the connection is not clear and fully understood, some research suggests that cardiovascular disease and stroke might be linked to the inflammation and infections that oral bacteria can cause. Oral problems such as the common painful toothache lead to lost work and school days; it also affects how speak, eat and breathe. Many clinical studies show that maintaining healthy teeth and gum is linked to longevity and higher quality of life in the elderly people.

A decrease in oral function as a result of aging has been shown to have major effects on mortality risk; it is a major risk factor for developing mal-nutrition. Oral frailty, a new concept introduced in Japan, is defined as a decrease in oral function, quite common in the old age group, and is often accompanied by a decrease in mental and physical functions. This is different from ' frailty ', a geriatric syndrome in the elderly population, characterized by diffuse weakness, unintentional weight loss, slow walking speed, inexplicable exhaustion, and very limited physical activity that is associated with adverse health outcomes. Perhaps, in the medical management of frailty, a dental professional should be part of the team.

To maintain and ensure oral health, it is important to brush your teeth two to three times a day for at least two minutes each time. You should floss daily and use mouthwash after brushing and flossing to remove any food particles. It is a good habit to replace your toothbrush every three to four months, or sooner. You should limit sugary food and drinks, and avoid tobacco use. Last but not least, schedule regular dental checkups and cleanings.

- Getting Adequate Sleep, 6 to 7 hours a day --- In the U.S., sleep deprivation is pretty common and its impact serious even though many people in our hectic, fast-pace society do not realize it, or simply ignore it, unaware of the potential adverse effects on our health and general well-being. It is a myth that it is ok to sleep five or fewer hours a night, because there is plenty of evidence to show that sleeping 5 hours or less a night consistently increases a person's risk considerably for adverse health consequences, including cardiovascular disease and early mortality. We all need adequate, quality sleep, which allows the body to rest and reset. This " down time " is necessary so that metabolic wastes can be eliminated optimally and effectively. It must be pointed out that during deep sleep, also known as rapid eye movement (REM) sleep, the body heals and recharges itself. Older people in general are light sleepers because they tend to spend less time in the deep stages of the sleep cycle. Moreover, getting a resfful night's sleep for them is often complicated by some physical ailments, aches and pains. Many of them can be suffering from sleep-disrupting side effects of medications they are taking.

In one very large sleep study, conducted at the University of California and involving one million participants, the researchers found that optimal sleep time for increased longevity is from six to seven hours for most people. The relationship between sleep and aging has been extensively studies, showing a number of age-related factors such as inflammation, elevated oxidative stress, mitochondrial decline and cellular senescence are found to be affected by sleep and sleep deprivation. Undoubtedly, sleep is essential for physical and mental well-being; it is one of the most important factors responsible for the maintenance of a healthy individual. It is known fact that sleep deprivation is one of the techniques used by the military establishment during interrogation of prisoners of war. It is undeniable that sleep represents a homeostatic need required for life!

The followings can be sleep-promoting:

If your sleep does not occur within 30 to 60 minutes of lying awake in bed, leave the bedroom and do something relaxing in another room.

Use the bedroom for sleeping and sex only.

It is important to go to bed and wake up at about the same time every day. With a regular sleep schedule, you can build up the natural sleep drive through a neuromodulator in your brain called adenosine.

Your bedroom should be cool, dark and uncluttered to create the optimal sleep environment. There is a false assumption that a warm bedroom is best for sleep. The National Sleep Foundation states that the ideal temperature for sleep is between 60 and 67 degrees Fahrenheit. Your brain responds better to cooler temperatures, making sleep easier for those who tend to have difficulty. It is even important to cover up any alarm clock that may emit light so you have a pitch-dark bedroom. This will enhance your natural circadian rhythms; upon arising, it is beneficial to get some exposure to sunlight to further strengthen the natural circadian rhythms.

To achieve further stimulus control, you need to avoid dramatic, violent and stressful entertainment with television, news program, movies and video games. It is not abnormal to awaken briefly during the night since sleep is polyphasic. It is imperative to follow the sleep hygiene so that you will be more productive and feeling better and refreshed the next day, with many more days to come.

Many people tend to minimize snoring during sleep, thinking that it is just annoying and not harmless. This assumption is potentially dangerous for your health because it can be a sign of sleep apnea. According to the American Sleep Apnea Association, about 22 million Americans suffer some form of sleep apnea. In fact, this number may be higher because this medical condition of sleep apnea is under-diagnosed.

Researchers at Harvard Medical School studied more than 2,800 individuals aged 65 and older to examine the relationship between sleep and their development of dementia over a period of at least five years. They found that individuals who slept fewer than five hours per night were twice as likely to develop dementia, and twice as likely to die. Another study by researchers in Europe, including France, the United Kingdom, the Netherlands, and Finland, who examined data from almost 8,000 participants. They found consistently that sleeping less than 6 hours a night was associated with a 30% increase in dementia risk compared to a normal sleep duration of seven hours. So, the theory is, and most experts believe, if you don't get adequate sleep, your brain won't have enough time to flush away beta amyloid and other toxic substances that accumulate during the day, resulting in dementia risk.

Ensuring six to seven hours of sleep should be a long-term goal and a desirable lifestyle for optimal physical and mental wellness. In fact, what you eat could have a major impact on this important aspect of your life. Here are some sleep-promoting foods before bed-time without resorting to melatonin supplement:

Almonds, pistachio nuts, strawberries, walnuts, cashews, tart cherry, edamame beans and tomatoes --- these are good sources of natural melatonin to help you get more and better sleep. Other foods include bananas, avocado, mushrooms and pomegranate due to their high levels of potassium.

Last but not least, lack of adequate sleep can have a negative effect on your immune system's ability to fight and prevent illness. Many people do not realize that your immune system works hard when you are asleep, cells are repaired, metabolic wastes are removed, and beneficial hormones like melatonin are released, etc. According to research, consistent sleep helps the immune system stay strong and finely-tuned, maintaining the balance and optimal functioning. In the short term, you may see side-effects of lack of adequate sleep like sleepiness, mood changes and memory problems and others; over the long term, you may experience potentially serious health concerns such as inflammation, increased risk of heart disease, weight gain and cognitive problems.

- **Sexual Activity and intimacy**--- More and more researches are showing that intimacy and sexual activity are beneficial to your health and general well-being. The landmark Masters and Johnson Study in 1986 links increased quality if life with the fulfillment of sexual desire. A 25-year study from Duke University found that the more sex you have, the longer you will live. Sexual health is important at any age and the desire for intimacy is timeless. Adults can remain sexually active regardless of age, and many people want and need to be close to others as they grow older. With aging, it is important and worthwhile for you to adapt sexual activity to accommodate physical conditions, health status and other changes. It is understandable that normal aging brings physical and physiological changes in both men and women, and these changes can affect the ability to have and enjoy sex.

There are different ways to have sex and be intimate: the expression of your sexuality can include many types of touch or stimulation. Sadly, some older adults have difficulty adapting to certain age-related changes and choose not to engage in sexual activity. And some are so set in their ways, and thus become " asexual". As you age, sex may not be the same as it was in your 20s, 30s and 40s, but it can still be fulfilling. As a matter of fact, the sex lives of older people should, more often than not, benefit from more experience and sexual confidence, and from relationships that have matured to a higher level of trust and intimacy. Ask yourself and your partner what is satisfying and mutually acceptable.

It is understandable that seniors face certain challenges to a satisfying sex life. Some health issues may get in the way, like vision and hearing---which often carry sexual cues---can fade with less acuity. Chronic illnesses can cause sexual problems, especially among older people. Just to name a few: joint pain due to arthritis; diabetes which can cause erectile dysfunction in some men and vaginal yeast infections in women; major surgeries for prostate in men and hysterectomy in women; cardiovascular disease with reduced arterial blood flow; loss of bladder control with leaking of urine; stroke with weakness and paralysis; and dementia. Here, people with dementia sometimes show increased interest in sex and physical closeness, but they may not be able to judge what is appropriate sexual behavior. Those with more advanced stage of dementia may not recognize their spouse or partner, but they still desire sexual contact and intimacy and may seek it with someone else.

A study in 2014 by the American Sexual Health Association showed that most people felt happy and healthy when their sex life was good and fulfilling. Don't assume that you are too old to have safe sex because age does not protect you from sexually transmitted diseases. Older people who are sexually active may be at risk for diseases such as syphilis, gonorrhea, chlamydial infection, genital herpes, hepatitis B, genital warts, trichomoniasis and HIV/AIDS. In fact, the number of seniors with HIV is on the rise, so are cases of STDs like chlamydia, herpes and hepatitis among seniors. Usually, it takes longer for older people to get aroused. That does not you are out of the game. The older couple need to be more creative and patient with an open mind. If your partner has more than one sexual partner, it is all the more important to use a condom for safe sex.

- Quit Smoking --- do yourself a big favor, and for your loved ones and friends around you, quit smoking cigarette. If you are not a smoker, it is highly advisable to avoid second-hand smoke. Most people are familiar with the increased risk of lung cancer associated with cigarette smoking, but unaware of, or ignoring, or not knowledgeable about the many other serious health consequences of smoking.

Life expectancy for habitual smokers is at least 10 years shorter than non-smokers because smokers face an increased risk for premature death. Furthermore, smokers have one thing in common: bad breath and smelly clothes. Smoking is the leading cause of preventable death in the U.S. – this is astounding for it represents one of every five deaths in the U.S. each year. This lamentable statistic does not even include the second-hand smoke which poses serious health hazard for other people around the smokers with thousands of deaths.

Cigarette smoking tends to accelerate the aging processes of the body: smokers are more likely to develop facial wrinkles and a haggard look. Apart from smokers themselves, many studies have shown that children of smoking parents have higher incidences of chronic obstructive pulmonary disease, such as bronchitis and emphysema. Smokers also have at least three times greater than non-smokers the chance of dying of a heart attack. Other long-term effects of smoking, regular or heavy, include loss of the abilities to smell and taste, eye cataracts and macular degeneration, and the yellowing of teeth and tooth decay.

Cigarette contains hundreds of harmful chemicals, and the most notorious one is nicotine, which is highly addictive and a powerful vaso-constrictor. Its property of vasoconstriction can increase blood pressure and reduce blood flow, raising the risk of stroke directly. Nicotine also heightens the rick for sudden death from ventricular arrhythmias, a serious and frightening condition which the heart does not beat normally, getting out of control.

The air-pollutants in the smoke and the toxic chemicals in the cigarette greatly increases the oxidative activities throughout the body, with the elevated levels of free radicals overwhelming and tilting the body's equilibrium. In other words, cigarette smoking is certainly the most insidious culprit for free-radical damages to the body, the brain in particular. The hundreds of free radicals in a puff of cigarette smoke also trigger inflammatory cells, adding more toxins and stress to the body. In fact, one can measure the damaged, oxidized fragments of DNA from cigarette smoking in the urine as 8-hydroxy-deoxyguanosine (8-OHdG).

So, if you want to have a healthy long lifespan, stay away from the vicious, bad habit of cigarette smoking and also stay away from people who smoke.

- **Alcohol Use and Your Health** --- Studies in Netherlands found statistically significant positive association between baseline alcohol intake and the probability of reaching 90 years or more in both men and women. Despite such findings and evidence that light to moderate consumption of alcohol can increase longevity, this is not free license to drink as much as you want. whether light to moderate alcohol intake is related to reduced mortality remains a subject of intense research and controversy. Research has clearly shown that regular alcohol consumption and binge drinking were not associated with longevity, and heavy drinkers have a higher risk of mortality. According to the Center for Disease Control and Prevention (CDC), excessive alcohol use is the fourth leading preventable cause of death in the U.S.

What is the definition of heavy drinking? It is defined as drinking eight drinks or more per week for women, and 15 drinks or more per week for men. In the U.S., a standard drink contains 0.6 ounces of pure alcohol in 12-ounces of beer, in 8-ounces of most liquor, and in 5-ounces of wine.

The risks of alcohol drinking can be divided into short-term and long-term ones. The short-term risks are most often the result of binge drinking (4 or more drinks for women during a single occasion and 5 or more drinks for men during a single occasion), and these short-term risks include injuries, motor vehicular accidents, drownings, falls, violence, inappropriate sexual behaviors, unintended pregnancy or sexually transmitted diseases, and alcohol poisoning.

The long-term health risks excessive alcohol use include:

+ High blood pressure, cardiovascular diseases, stroke, liver disease and digestive problems such as ulcers.

+ Cancers of the liver and the digestive tract such as the esophagus, colon and rectum.

+ Learning and memory problems

+ Social issues including family and legal problems, and job-related problems

+ Mental health problems, including depression and anxiety.

+ Alcohol addiction

+ Malnutrition and vitamin deficiency

+ Immune system dysfunction

Over time, the frontal lobe of the brain can be permanently damaged, leading to Wernicke-Korsakoff Syndrome, a degenerative brain disorder.

There are some people who should not drink any alcohol at all due to certain health/medical conditions; it is important to consult your physicians for clear directions. For example, many older people are taking multiple prescriptions, some of which may interact with alcohol. Even some over-the-counter medications cannot be taken in the presence of alcohol. As a caveat, a large study by the University of Pennsylvania recently published in the ' Nature Communications ' journal with over 36,000 adult participants found that even moderate amount of alcohol consumption, the so-called healthy drinking, can alter the cellular structures of the brain reducing their capacity to function. The researchers discovered that even low level of alcohol use was associated with dwindled volume of white and gray matter, resulting in brain atrophy. This study was groundbreaking because of the huge sample size, which provided an unprecedented amount of data for analyses.

- Social Connections --- staying socially engaged and connected is important for a long, meaningful life because social isolation can often lead to chronic illnesses or exacerbation thereof and depression. A long list of friends may add years to your life. Tel Aviv University researchers followed 820 adults for 20 years and found that those with the most social support lived the longest. Friendship is the key in Sardinia, Italy, a tiny Mediterranean island with a large centenarian population, one of the five blue zones in the world.

  Researchers at Duke-NUS' Center for Aging Research and Education (CARE) in Singapore found that lonely older adults can expect to live a shorter life than their peers who don't perceive themselves as lonely. This and other similar studies is timely because the stay-at-home and physical distancing measures and mandates since the start of the COVID-19 pandemic have only intensified concern for the mental and physical well-being of older people isolated or quarantined. Unfortunately, this challenging global event of COVID-19 has left pretty much everyone on the planet feeling more lonely and isolated than ever.

  In the U.S., at least one in ten Americans live alone, according to the most recent statistics, and many are at risk for loneliness. Many of these lonely individuals are older, and the trend will continue because the geriatric population is the fastest growing segment of the world. A close friend is hard to find nowadays, but you may find that, as you get older, friends are often more difficult to keep. Sadly, it is becoming increasingly clear the average American adult has fewer friends and is lonelier than ever. According to the May 2021 American Perspectives Survey, just under half (49%) of American adults report only having three or fewer good friends. That's a big leap in comparison to 1990, when only 27% of Americans said they had three or fewer close friends. Someone might wonder: " What is the big deal, anyway?" We, humans, are social creatures by our very nature. Loneliness or social isolation is bad in many ways, and is hazardous to your health. For an older adult, it impacts more than just the lifespan; it also adversely affects your quality of life due to higher risk of functional disability.

Psychosocial researches have shown that lonely people experience more insomnia, more depression, more susceptible to infections due to less effective immune system. Lonely people face greater risk of premature death from all illnesses. People who have mutually caring interpersonal relationships enjoy increased sense of well-being, both mentally and physically, display greater emotional resilience, and live longer and happier lives.

Social isolation is undeniably unhealthy because it causes a stress response in the body, leading to chronic inflammation. Over time, chronic loneliness may raise your risk of becoming seriously ill and development of cancer, according to some research conducted at Yale Medicine. A study published in the Journal of Antioxidants and Redox Signaling, the long-term inflammation caused by loneliness may represent a key mechanism in the development of loneliness-associated chronic diseases such as atherosclerosis, cancer, coronary artery disease and neurodegenerative disorders including dementia. A study published in March 2022 in JAMA Network Open suggested that social isolation and loneliness in elderly women in the United States were associated with a 27% higher risk for severe cardiovascular disease. There were approximately 60,000 women aged 65-99 participated in this significant study.

Each of us came to this world through the body of another being. Every person was once part of his or her mother, connected to her body and contained and nurtured within it. We all bear the sign of that wonderful and blessed connection --- the umbilicus (navel). This is a sign of where we came from, and a membership card in the human club. As of 2020, the numbers of adults aged over 30 made up half the total global population, marking the beginning of an increasingly aging world. As a consequence, loneliness among the elderly has become an issue of social and public health concern, and will only worsen if we continue to ignore and not treat it preemptively and proactively. LONELINESS IS A DISEASE OF DISCONNECTION !

- **Spirituality and Longevity** --- A growing body of scientific studies has demonstrated a consistently positive association between religious-spiritual involvement and beneficial effects on physical health, culminating with increased longer lifespan. This protective effect on the mortality risk is not only statistically significant but also clinically relevant. A recent health letter from Mayo Clinic suggested that one of the best ways to improve your chances to live longer is to recognize the value of spirituality in your life. The Mayo Clinic health center advised that you should nurture your spirit, no matter what you call your source of inspiration.

Until recently, very little attention is paid to the emotional component of our health; stress can become an important factor in many illnesses. There is a plethora of evidence that negative emotions and stress do impact our life and health adversely. Even though the traditional medical community has been taking a more cautious approach on this subject; nowadays, the door is widely opened for the holistic approach, including spirituality and faith. A new field of medical science has started, called Psychoneuroimmunology, which studies how your mind influences your health and how social and psychological factors, such as faith, affect the immune and nervous systems. Spirituality is a rather broad term that includes a sense of connection to some being bigger and higher than oneself. The meaning of spirituality has developed over time and different connotations can be found alongside each other.

Traditionally, spirituality refers to a religious process of re-formation, oriented at "the image of God" as exemplified by the founders and sacred texts of the world religions. The term, spirituality, was used within Early Christianity oriented toward the Holy Spirit; it was then broadened during the Late Middle Ages to include mental aspects of life. In modern times, the term, spirituality spreads to other religious traditions, including subjective experiences of a sacred dimension, often separate from organized religious institutions.

The word ' spirit ' is derived from the Latin spiritus, meaning ' soul, courage, vigor breath '. Aging and spirituality are interwoven in a mystical and awe-inspiring way. Spirituality provides shelter for the aging and at the same time it makes the aging process a wonderful journey! In the confines of spirituality, the fear of aging will disappear. The cells of your body will benefit and you will have a greater sense of wellness. Studies have shown that spirituality strengthen the mind. When the mind becomes strong, your body follows suit. In fact, an individual can become spiritual non-religiously, without belonging to any specific religious entity. Spirituality widens the horizon, and helps you to pursue and understand the meaning and purpose of your life.

I believe that one is more than just one's own physical body, and there is more to life than the material world. We are actually spiritual beings inhabiting the material/physical forms. Spirituality deals with the non-physical parts of you, such as the way you think and feel. It often points to the fundamental human quest for understanding the ultimate truth of human existence. While its concept is personal, private and individual, religion brings together people of similar beliefs and similar spirituality. In fact, spiritual experiences are surprisingly common, even among those who describe themselves as non-religious.

Many studies in social and psychological sciences have demonstrated that religious people are happier, healthier, recovering better after traumas, and living longer than non-religious people. Those active in their religion report greater social support through their organizational establishments. They tend to live longer with longer survival rates after cardiac surgeries probably due to strength, comfort and hope from their faith. Furthermore, according to researchers, spiritual and religious people are more likely to have healthier lifestyles with positive outlook and harmonious family life. In general, they suffer less from anxiety and depression, less prone to suicide, less likely to smoke, and less likely to abuse drugs and alcohol.

Most of the research in social studies have shown that people who attend church regularly live about 7 years longer than those who are non-religious and do not attend church.

Religion is usually practiced within a fellowship of kindred spirits, sharing one another's burdens, reaching out to those in need and offering assistance when possible, including friendship and companionship. Dr. David Koenig of Duke University Medical Center, as founder and Director of the Center for the Study of Religion, Spirituality and Health has written more than 35 books and hundreds of articles on how religious beliefs and observance positively influence our mental and physical well-beings. He states that " religious attendance produces positive social, psychological and behavioral consequences ".

Duke University studied 4,000 people for four years and found that those who attended church weekly had a 28 percent lower mortality rate overall when compared to those who did not belong to a church community. Other factors considered by the researchers in this study included income, education, chronic illnesses, health habits, exercise, smoking, alcohol consumption, body fat and psychological status. However, none of these explained the results. Church attendance seemed to be an independent predictor, and the strongest predictor of longevity.

It is important for us to keep an open mind, whether you are a believer or not; there is a saying that "absence of evidence is NOT evidence of absence".

The followings are more things you can do as a non-dietary approach to longevity:

- Washing your hands when necessary and recommended for at least 20 seconds with appropriate soap or cleaners. According to a study by the World Health Organization, the simple act of hand-washing could save more lives worldwide than any vaccine or other medical intervention.

- Taking more vacation. According to the analyses of the famous Framingham Heart Study, they found that the more frequent men took vacation, the longer they lived.
- Don't retire from life when you are retired from your career. It should be the time for you to find and learn new interest without time constraint. Retirement does not mean resting and staying still. Be a volunteer in your community or share your experiences.
- Use safety gears. Accidents are one of the leading causes of death in the U.S. Seatbelts reduce the chances of death or serious injuries in a car wreck by 50%. Wear a helmet because many deaths from bicycle accidents are caused by traumas to the head. If you are swimming in the open water at the beach, wear the floatation safety vest even if you know how to swim.
- Take the stairs if you can. Researchers from the University of Geneva calculated that many people with a sedentary lifestyle or job, simply taking the stairs was enough physical activity to burn body fat and lower blood pressure and enough to cut their risk of an early death by 15%.
- Get a Pet. Pets are not just great companions to beat loneliness, they can actually help you meet human pals, too. One study shows that people who own dogs are more likely to know the folks in the neighborhood. They also get interactions and exchange advice with people they meet through their pets. According to a recent study published by the National Library of Medicine, researchers explored the influence that pets had on adults who were dealing with Alzheimer's disease over a five-year period. The results revealed substantial positive effects pets have on their human friends. The data also conclude that pets may help everyday activity and actually slow down the progression of Alzheimer's. They truly make good company, and encourage you to get outside in the fresh air to have a chance to socialize. It is undeniable that an increase in physical

activity can benefit cognitive health. They, furthermore, give you the responsibility as their caregivers.

Many studies have demonstrated that having a pet is beneficial for your overall physical and mental wellbeing. Individuals with a dog live longer than those who do not have a dog, according to research data recorded in the journal of Circulation in 2019.

Having friends including pets is undoubtedly good for a person's health; indeed, loneliness and isolation can increase a person's risk of premature death, increase the risk of dementia, cause anxiety and depression, and more. The human-animal bond has been shown to decrease blood pressure and stress, and slow cognitive decline. We know that stress can adversely affect cognitive function, and the stress-buffering effects of pet ownership have been proven in many studies. In the Health and Retirement study, the research team studied over 1,300 people with an average of 65. Over 60% of the participants were pet-owners. Multiple cognitive tests were given to the participants, and the team developed a composite cognitive score for each person who took the tests which included subtraction, numerical counting and word recall. The findings were twofold: For pet-owners over a period of six years, their cognitive scores decreased at a slower rate than participants without pets. Secondly, pet owners had a composite cognitive score that was 1.2 points higher on average at six years compared to people that did not own a pet.

- Take control of your medical care. Not understanding your medications and treatments can raise your risk of death. Studies have shown that patients who do not ask questions or do not understand their medical conditions are at an increased risk of complication and death. It is important for you to take time to research and learn about your

- medical conditions and diagnoses because it can save your life. Nowadays, the digital technology with Internet makes it easy for anyone to search for information.
- Get yourself tested. You need to be proactive, making a commitment to keep up with the preventative care and screening plans you have with your physician. When an illness or a medical condition is detected early, the rate of success and cure is the highest.
- Keep your brain busy. More and more research show that a healthy brain into old age depends on intellectual stimulations. A busy brain is good for longevity. So, take some classes, learn new things and stay smart.
- Your home environment and its design can affect your longevity. Many long-living people live in home environments that kind of nudge them unconsciously toward healthier behaviors, like moving more. Older people tend to spend most of the time indoors. For example, people tend to eat past the point of fullness when they are watching TV, and it is a healthy idea to have the television away from the kitchen. With such arrangement, you are not only less likely to snack mindlessly, but also you have an opportunity to get up and walk for your snack.

With a shoe rack by the front door, you will more likely to take off your shoes when you get home, a common practice among people in Okinawa, Japan. Studies show that 28 percent of shoes carry fecal bacteria. Sharing a meal with others at home leads you to eat more slowly, allowing adequate time for the fullness signal to reach the brain. Socializing and eating with family and friends at home is a prominent feature on the Blue Zones.

For older individuals, incorporating low couches and chairs throughout your home is a good way to steer clear of a fall that could compromise your longevity. It is estimated that 25 percent of older Americans suffer a fall each year, and it is one of the leading causes of hospitalization. Make your bathroom safe to prevent slips and trips by laying slip-resistant mats on the floor, or installing slip-proof tiles, and adding grab-bars to the walls of the bath-tub. Ideally, installing a walk-in tub to take a shower with a bench so that you do not need to climb over the ledge to get into it. Make certain that there is sufficient lighting, including natural sunlight. Last but not least, install electronic emergency alarm with a pull string in case of emergency!

Nutrition and longevity, the dietary approach to a healthy, long lifespan:

The famous quote by Greek physician Hippocrates "Let food be thy medicine, and let medicine be thy food" has stood the test of time for over 2000 years. This is perhaps one of the best-known quotes on diet and health attributed to Hippocrates, the physician-philosopher in Ancient Greece, and is considered the father of Modern Medicine. This universally succinct phrase points to the importance of our daily food choices, and its relevance is stronger than ever. Research has shown that the effect of a proper, healthy diet is much stronger on the inner workings of our cells than the intake of drugs, especially in the cases of type-2 diabetes, stroke and cardiovascular disease. Many studies of therapeutic nutrition suggest that nutrition has a greater impact on aging and metabolic health than medications. It is a fact that what we eat affects our health because food can dramatically influence or impact many of the processes operating within our cells.

Hippocrates held and believed that reason, logic and science are central to the practice of medicine. He further reminded healers to treat patients with respect, to listen to their patients, and not to try to enforce their conclusions, sometimes to the detriment of healing. ' Do No Harm " is indeed a maxim! The Hippocrates diet uses only plant-based foods, usually uncooked because heating destroys enzymes found in living food. The vegetables should ne fresh, organic and raw, and the fruits should be ripe when harvested in order to optimally improve energy and strengthen the immune system.

An educated and conscientious intake of foods, including fluids, is critical and important to have a balanced diet leading to a long, healthy lifespan. First and foremost is water to stay hydrated:

- There are plenty of lifestyle adjustments you can make to slow down the process of aging. Some adjustments are bigger than others, but drinking adequate fluid is a small and easy way for you to lead to longevity. Most of us tend to take water for granted because it is so freely and readily available everywhere. Ironically, many people are not drinking enough water, and chronic dehydration is actually quite common. Nowadays, with the constant advertisements and ubiquitous sensual bombardments about manufactured beverages such as beer, mixed coffee, sodas including the diet version, and juices, most people are paying less and less attention to simple, pure water. In fact, most of those commercial beverages advertised contain dehydrating ingredients which deplete the water content of the body, though unintentionally.

The human body is about 70% water, whereas the human brain is at least 75% water and is very sensitive to any degree of dehydration at cellular levels. Many people do not realize that water is not just a simple, inert substance; it is life-giving and life-sustaining. Each cell of human body is about 75% water, which is important in biochemical reactions and in the production of electrical energy for brain functions, including thinking. One of the first signs of dehydration is brain fog --- being unable to concentrate and having difficulty remembering things.

To prevent dehydration, you must drink water regularly every day; the human body does not store water for us to draw from in case of dehydration. According to a study published in the journal Mechanism of Ageing and Development, dehydration is something that affects 20 to

30% of older people. According to Harvard Health, most healthy people should aim to drink around six cups of water a day. Research has suggested that there is a link between dehydration, higher mortality and disability in older people. Build a healthy habit of drinking fluid gradually throughout your day; however, you can drink too much water if you suffer from health conditions such as thyroid disease, kidney, heart and liver problems. If so, your water intake is something you must discuss with your physician.

As we get older, we lose the sharpness, acuity and precision of our senses including hearing, vision, smell and thirst. Due to the gradual loss of thirst, more and more old people fail to drink water adequately. This phenomenon has profound, detrimental effects on the elderly both physically and mentally. To make the matter worse, people often confuse the sensation of thirst with the feeling of hunger. So, instead of drinking water, which is essentially an appetite suppressant, they eat foods adding more calories to their weight and become more dehydrated. Studies by Phillips and Associates have shown that after 24 hours of water deprivation, the elderly participants still do not realize or recognize that they are thirsty. Other studies published in the Lancet, a renowned British medical journal, have supported the conclusion that the thirst mechanism is gradually lost in the elderly with aging.

An important scientific paper by Ephraim Katchalski-Katzir of the Weitzmann Institute demonstrated that proteins and enzymes function more efficiently in solutions of lower viscosity, i.e. they need adequate water in their immediate milieu to work optimally. The most significant complication and consequence of dehydration is the loss of the necessary essential amino acids in the production od neuro-transmitters. Therefore, chronic dehydration can disrupt neuronal function and cause neurological damage to the brain because raw materials become less available for the brain to make neurotransmitters.

The body and brain are maintained on a fine-tuned system of homeostasis, and dehydration throws the balance off. When necessary nutrients like salt become too concentrated in the blood, one can experience 'altered mental state' and if dehydration continues without treatment, it can lead to seizures. Furthermore, chronic dehydration is associated with shrinking brain tissue and reduced brain volume, according to the findings of studies published in JAMA Psychiatry. Many consumers are so used to the different flavors and additives in the beverages they drink every day, a cup of simple, clean and pure water is the last thing they want to drink on the list. It will be more enticing and nutritious adding a piece of lemon to your water.

Be A Fish Lover and an educated seafood consumer about the levels of mercury in certain fish. Fish and their omega-3 fatty acids are key to longevity. For a healthy, long lifespan, inclusion of fish in your diet regularly is more than a recommendation, it is a must! Fish and seafood are an important feature in the Blue Zone and Mediterranean diets.

Fatty fish, seaweed and marine algae are good sources of the "good fat", and the omega-3 fatty acids in fish like salmon, tuna, sardines and mackerel can help lower your risk of dying, according to a 2013 study published in the Annals of Internal Medicine. Researchers from the Harvard School of Public health found that people with high levels of omega-3 fatty acids in their blood --- levels maintained by eating fish at least twice a week --- lived for 2.2 years longer, on average, than people with low levels of omega-3 fatty acids. But eating fish can do more than extend your life --- it can improve the quality of life because omega-3 fatty acids can help you to fight different diseases to live a better, healthier life.

There are three main forms of omega-3 fatty acids, DHA (docosahexaenoic acid) and EPA (eicosapentaenoic acid) come from fish; ALA (alpha linolenic acid) tend to be plant-based foods. Such as nuts and seeds. Some of the best plant-sources of ALA include walnuts, kidney beans, edamame, chia seeds, flaxseeds and hemp seeds. It is not just the omega-3FAs that play a role in promoting health benefits, but the ratio between omega-3FAs and omega-6FAs. Researchers have found that a high consumption of omega-6 in relation to omega-3FAs is linked to unhealthy inflammation and an increased risk of diseases. Those who follow a Western diet high in processed, fried and greasy foods are typically eating too much omega-6FAs relative to omega-3FAs; this can lead to various health problems.

Let us look at some of the health benefits from eating fish and maintaining a high blood level of omega-3 fatty acids:

1. Omega-3 FAs are good for your heart, many studies have shown. Eating at least two servings a week, fish high in omega-3FAs can reduce one's risk for heart attack and strokes, according to a 2011 review of more than 250 studies published in the journal of American College of Cardiology.
2. Fish help reduce prostate cancer risk. Men who regularly eat fish have a lower risk of prostate cancer, according to a 2011 study published in the journal of Nutrigenetics and Nutrigenomics. Research from the University of California, San Francisco, looked at more than 900 men and found that those who had the highest intake of omega-3FAs were at a 63 percent lower risk of developing aggressive prostate

cancer. One of the explanations is the anti-angiogenic property of omega-3FAs to fight the cancer.
3. Eating fish with high levels of omega-3FAs may help to prevent breast cancer, according to a 2013 review in the journal of BMJ. Researchers from Zhejiang University, China analyzed the results of 26 studies involving more than 800,000 participants and found those who ate at least 0.1 gram of omega-3 FAs daily had aa 5% lower risk of breast cancer than those who did not eat omega-3 FAs. The higher the levels of omega-3 FAs, the lower the risk of breast cancer. The Singapore Chinese Health Study examined the HEALTH OF 35,298 WOMEN AND FOUND THAT eating 3 ounces of fish every day was associated with a 26% reduced risk of breast cancer, while the EPIC study showed that eating more than three ounces of fish daily was associated with a 31% decreased risk of colon cancer.
4. Omega-3 FAs in fish help treat autoimmune diseases, most likely the positive effect is augmented by other nutrients in the fish. Patients with Rheumatoid Arthritis, psoriasis and other inflammation AND AUTOIMMUNE disorders would benefit from regularly eating fish or taking a fish oil supplements, according to a 2002 study published in the journal of the American College of Nutrition. Researchers from the Center for Genetics, Nutrition and Health in Washington, D.C. found that patients with autoimmune diseases who regularly eat fish and/or took fish oil supplement did better with treatments than their counterparts who did not consume fish in their diet. The patients with high levels of omega-3 FAs showed decreased disease activity and required less use of the anti-inflammatory drugs.
5. In the Women's Health Study of 38,022 middle-aged women, Harvard researchers found that those who

consumed one or more servings of fatty fish per week over a 10-year period had a 42 percent decreased risk of developing age-related macular degeneration (AMD), which is the most common cause of vision loss among people aged 50 and over. A large meta-analysis involving 128,988 people across eight different studies in Iceland, the Netherlands, United States, and Australia showed that eating, ranging from once a month to three to four times per week, was associated with a decreased risk of AMD by 24 percent.

6. According to the researchers at Barcelona Beta Brain Research Center in Barcelona, Spain, they studied middle-aged adults who were at higher genetic risk for the development of Alzheimer's disease, that is, they had two ApoE4 alleles, and found that those individuals with a high intake of DHA exhibited more resistance to pathologic structural changes in their brains. Their brain scans revealed mush less atrophy and cortical thinning on neuro-imaging. In 2009, scientists at Sweden's Gothenburg University reported that 15-years-old boys and girls who ate fish at least twice a week scored higher on intelligence tests than their non-fish-eating peers.

Studies have demonstrated that low levels of DHA in the hippocampus may have a role in the cognitive decline in the elderly and in Alzheimer's patients. In fact, Alzheimer's patients generally exhibit lower levels of DHA in their plasma and brain. Epidemiologically, researchers have noticed that increasing DHA via dietary intake of seafood can reduce the risk of Alzheimer's disease with less cell death and apoptosis, and enhanced signaling pathways. This is probably due to the ability of DHA to increase the production of anti-inflammatory molecules and to reduce the viscosity of the blood, thus improving blood flow and preventing strokes.

According to recent Harvard studies, fish is the single most important for cognitive health, especially in Alzheimer's disease, from the standpoint of dietary factor.

The brain is about 60 percent fat, and most of that is DHA, docosahexaenoic acid, which is a polyunsaturated omega-3 fatty acid. DHA is vital and extremely crucial for optimal functioning of the brain , and is very important in the development of the fetal brain and spinal cord. Let us look at some of the vital roles played by these specialized fats:

1. They serve as rich sources of energy.
2. They facilitate the absorption of fat-soluble vitamins and important nutrients including vitamins A,D,E,K, and carotenoids such as lutein, lycopene and beta-carotene.
3. They serve as essential building blocks for cell membranes and plasma membranes.
4. They provide insulation and protective linings for vital organs, e.g. lung surfactant.
5. They are required for the production of bile which aids in proper digestion.
6. They serve as structural component of myelin sheath of the neurons, facilitating effective neuronal communications and signaling.

Currently, the biggest nutritional deficiency in the Western countries is the low intake of omega-3 polyunsaturated fatty acids in the form of fresh fish, not the popular fried variety. Most of the healthy, fatty fish are common, readily available, and safe in terms of their mercury levels; just to name a few: salmon, sardines, mackerel, pollock, trout, anchovy, catfish, herring and many others. For the regular seafood (Fish) consumers, you must be cautious and educated about the levels of mercury, which is neurotoxic and dangerous to your health. The U.S. Food and Drug Administration (FDA) has issued guidelines in this regard for the consumers. So, not all fish are created equal, and some of them can be harmful to your health due to their higher neurotoxic mercury content. Fish with potentially high mercury levels include, but not limited to:

- Shark
- Tilefish
- Marlin
- Swordfish
- King Mackerel
- Orange Roughy
- Tuna

Green leafy vegetables and fruits:

In general, a Western diet seems to be deficient in green leafy vegetables and fruits, which are a staple food in the five Blue Zones. With a plant-based diet, it naturally comes with plenty of fibers. More and more research continue to prove the link between eating a high-fiber diet and living a long life.

One study published in JAMA Internal Medicine demonstrated that diets rich in dietary fiber can reduce the risk of death from cardiovascular, respiratory, and infectious diseases. A meta-analysis of 17 studies published in the American Journal of Epidemiology found that for every 10 grams of fiber consumed, it reduced the mortality risk by 10% among the participants. A 2019 study in the Lancet concluded that diets high in fiber (consuming between 25 and 29 grams of fiber a day) cut the risk of coronary heart disease, stroke, type-2 diabetes, colorectal cancer, and also significantly helped lowering total cholesterol, blood pressure, and even body weight

The Mediterranean Diet:

It is the diet, fresh and colorful, followed by residents of the Mediterranean, which consists of the densest population of people who live to be over 100. In 2018, 2910, 2020 and 2022, it was ranked as the best diet by U.S. News and World Report, ideal for heart protection, weight regulation, cancer reduction and mental health. Mediterranean diet is about whole, unprocessed natural foods; it is not about a specific food per se, but about the overall style of eating.

It is a way of eating based on traditional cuisine of countries bordering the Mediterranean Sea. It is typically high in vegetables, fruits, whole grains, beans, nuts and seeds along with olive oil. It is usually low in the consumption of meat and alcohol. Undoubtedly, it is good for the heart and brain; many studies have shown that Mediterranean diet is strongly linked to longevity. A Harvard study published in the BMJ suggests that this diet may also help protect your telomeres. Telomere is considered to be one of the biomarkers of aging; shorter telomeres are associated with a lower life expectancy and higher rates of developing age-related chronic diseases.

Interest in the diet began in the 1950s when it was noted that heart disease was not as common in Mediterranean countries as it was in the U.S. A study published in the New England Journal of Medicine has shown that Mediterranean diet can help reduce the risk of heart attack, strokes and death related to heart problems by 30 percent. In a study on women, those who closely followed a Mediterranean diet had a lower BMI and smaller waist and thighs than those who adhered to the diet the least. A 2016 review of 18 studies in 'Frontier in Nutrition' found that eating Mediterranean diet was associated with less cognitive decline, reduced the risk of Alzheimer's disease, and better memory and executive functions. Additional research in the journal likened the diet's effects to reducing the brain's age by five years. The diet is high in antioxidants and it provides anti-inflammatory properties; it is also packed with fiber, a nutrient known for keeping you full and your intestinal tract lubricated for elimination of metabolic wastes from the body.

According to the findings from recent studies, researchers have found a link between eating a Mediterranean-style diet and delayed onset of Parkinson's disease. The delayed onset of this neurodegenerative disorder can be as much as 17 years. In other words, the neuro-scientists support that adherence to the Mediterranean diet can reduce the incidence and delay the progression of neurodegenerative diseases such as Alzheimer's and Parkinson's. It is not surprising from the plethora of supportive and encouraging evidence that Mediterranean diet is now considered an important modifiable factor in Alzheimer's disease. In a 2013 study of 550 people aged between 55 and 80 by researchers in Spain, the participants were randomly assigned either a low-fat diet plan or a Mediterranean diet. The followed their assigned diets for 6.5 years; the follow-up results showed that those who ate a Mediterranean diet scored the highest on cognitive tests.

A 5-year-long study of 960 adults aged 81 and older who were dementia-free at the start of the study was published in the journal of the Alzheimer's Association, the researchers found that those who followed the MIND diet to the letter (created by Rush University in Chicago and short for Mediterranean-Dash Intervention for Neurodegenerative Diseases) dramatically reduced their risk of Alzheimer's disease by as much as 53 percent. For those participants who did not adhere to the MIND diet whole-heartedly still reduced their risk of the disease by 35 percent.

Other researchers in several recent studies found that the brains of healthy, middle-aged individuals who faithfully followed the Mediterranean diet had less atrophy on the MRI brain scans and less accumulation of the beta-amyloid protein than people who did not follow the specific diet regimen. Most experts and researchers seem to agree that the Mediterranean diet is able to positively influence inflammation and oxidative stress in the brain, of course the body also,, lowering their levels and reducing the formation of plaques and tangles that cause damages to the neurons.

According to a recent study published by the University of Edinburgh, the Mediterranean diet is also linked to better thinking skills later in life, keeping you mentally sharp. The researchers tested over 500 people all at the age of 79 and without dementia. The participants completed numerous tests to evaluate their problem solving, thinking speed, memory and word knowledge along with MRI scans of the brains. The results of this study revealed that people who adhered to the Mediterranean diet had higher scores for cognitive functions. In particular, the individual diet components that stood out to the researchers were higher consumption of leafy green vegetables and lower consumption of red meat.

Researchers at the German Center for Neurodegenerative Diseases in Bonn studied the brain scans of more than 500 older adults who ate a Mediterranean diet and found that they were less likely to show brain shrinkage and had lower blood levels of the abnormal protein, amyloids. Following conscientiously a Mediterranean diet could help slow down the progression of Alzheimer's disease and prevent cognitive decline, as they reported these findings in the medical journal ' Neurology '.

Let us look at some of the components in the Mediterranean diet:

- **Green leafy vegetables** --- Many studies have consistently shown that eating more green leafy vegetables is important for healthy aging. According to researchers from the University of Illinois at Urbana-Champaign and the University of Georgia, Lutein, a carotenoid with powerful antioxidant property found in green leafy vegetables, may protect against cognitive decline with aging. Studies by researchers from Rush University, Chicago and Tufts Human Nutrition Research Center in Boston were published in the journal Neurology; they found that eating one serving of green leafy vegetables is associated with slower age-related cognitive decline. The participants were 81 years on average and followed over a period of five years.

   Foods high in lutein are common and readily available; these include kale, spinach, Brussels sprouts, Swiss chard, broccoli, asparagus, arugula, etc. There are many healthy nutrients and bio-actives in green leafy vegetables besides lutein, such as vitamin K, nitrate, folate, alpha-tocopherol, beta-carotene and flavonoids. However, lutein accumulates in brain tissues and in the eyes, and this allows researchers to easily measure lutein levels.

For healthy aging and longevity, consuming green leafy vegetables is one of the non-negotiables! Colorful leafy vegetables are great sources of polyphenols, which are powerful antioxidants and anti-inflammatories. Many studies including the one conducted at the University of Barcelona have shown that polyphenols, bioactive compounds from plants, could help reduce the risk of cognitive decline and bolster longevity. Population projections by many researchers including the World Health Organization of the United Nations include a sharp increase in the prevalence of dementia worldwide as the oldest age groups continue to grow in number. Decline in cognitive abilities is the central feature, one of the most feared conditions of aging.

- Adding olive oil --- It is packed with healthy fats, nutrients and antioxidants, and is a crucial part and a vital ingredient of the Mediterranean diet. Olive oil has a long history dating back centuries. The Ancient Greeks thought of the olive as a 'sacred fruit' and were the first to refine olives into oil. No wonder Greece is the world's leading olive oil consumer. The Romans associated olive oil with elite society, consuming it, the golden liquid, to extend life. While olive oil has been popular in the Mediterranean for thousands of years, it did not gain footing in the U.S. until the '90s.

  Adding olive oil, according to new research at the Harvard TH Chan School of Public Health. The researchers studied the diet of 60,582 women and 31,801 men from 1900-2018. During the 28 years of research, those who said they consumed more than a half tablespoon of olive oil daily had a 19% lower risk of all causes of death, as well as 19% lower risk of cardiovascular disease, compared to those who rarely or never used olive oil.

Oleic acid, the main monounsaturated fatty acid of olive oil, may have anti-cancer properties, according to some studies. People in the Mediterranean countries have a lower risk of some cancers; many researchers believe that oleic acid in olive oil may be the reason. Their lower incidence of colorectal cancer, breast and prostate cancer is probably due to the high consumption of olive oil, which exerts beneficial actions and effects in terms of cancer prevention.

Of course, one must pay attention to their overall diet quality and lifestyle to achieve healthy longevity. The key point is to add olive oil into the diet as a substitution of other unhealthy fats, which seem to be ubiquitous in the Western world, especially fast foods. By the way, consumption of olive oil is not associated with weight gain and obesity, according to many studies, even though olive oil contains fat. But unlike butter and lard, olive oil does not have fats that are solid at room temperature. The monounsaturated fatty acids in olive oil are healthy fats with its ph4enolic compounds, antioxidants, and fat-derived beneficial molecules like tocopherols.

According to a recent study published in the Journal of the American College of Cardiology, researchers found that people with a higher intake of olive oil are "more likely to experience positive health outcomes, including a reduced risk of early death. ". One of the interesting properties of extra virgin olive oil is that it can withstand rather high frying temperatures, with a smoke point between 325 and 375 degrees, favorable as compared to most other common cooking oils with lower smoke points. Chemically, when oil breaks down at certain temperature, it can release carcinogenic compounds such as aldehydes and lipid peroxides.

- **Drinking wine** --- Sardinians are famous for their daily consumption of the regional red wine called Cannonau. Most people in the Blue Zones drink alcohol moderately and regularly. The key is to drink one or two glasses a day with friends and meals, not save it up all week and have a binge at one sitting on one day. Consuming the wine with foods can help the body absorb more of the flavonoids, the strong antioxidants. The Sardinian shepherds often walk up to five miles a day tending to their flocks. According to a study completed by the European Society of Cardiology, moderate wine drinking and regular exercise is a healthy combination that can protect against cardiovascular disease.

The health benefits of red wine have been studied in many modern biochemical research; the scientists have shown that a moderate consumption of red wine have positive, beneficial impact on endothelial function, dyslipidemia, hypertension and metabolic disorders due to its antioxidant properties.

Resveratrol is the polyphenol found in the skin of grapes is known to protect the body against cellular damages. It can also be found in other plant foods, such as apples, blueberries, plums, and peanuts. Research has found that resveratrol can activate the longevity-related protein, Sirtuin-1, and improve the function of the mitochondria. According to a study conducted at New York's Litwin-Zucker Research Center, resveratrol can combat the formation of plaque that is found in the brains of dementia patients.

In another study published in the journal of Prevention of Alzheimer's disease, participants who consumed alcohol at least once a week, had significantly better cognitive function in old age than those who did not drink at all. Red wine may be the elixir to help us live a long life with its many potential health benefits, but it is far from a cure-all.

The following is something the moderate red wine drinkers should be aware of:

The World Heart Federation (WHF) states in a new policy brief in January of 2022 that " the widely held notion that consuming small to moderate amounts of alcohol is good to cardiovascular health is not supported by data ". The organization further indicates that the evidence is clear that any level of drinking can contribute to a loss of a healthy life. According to the WHF in their recent brief, over the past several decades, the prevalence of cardiovascular disease has nearly doubled, and alcohol has played a major role in the incidence of much of it.

The World Heart Federation advised that one should never under-estimate the harm and danger of alcohol consumption. In fact, following a recent report of the Lancet based on the Global Burden of Disease, the WHF concluded that " there is no safe level of alcohol consumption ".

In 2019, nearly 2.4 million deaths were attributed to alcohol, accounting for 4.3 percent of all deaths globally. WHF claims that even small amounts of alcohol have been shown to increase the risk for cardiovascular disease, atrial fibrillation, coronary disease, stroke, hypertensive heart disease, and aneurysm.

After all, we must be responsible for our own health and be knowledgeable of what we eat and drink. Nobody knows your body better than yourself while keeping an open mind. Researchers at the University of Texas looked at study participants aged 55 to 65 over a 20-year period, and took into account of other factors such as socioeconomic status, physical activities, friends and social support. They found that mortality rates were the highest for those who had never consumed alcohol of any kind, lower for the heavy drinkers, and mortality rates were the lowest for moderate drinkers who enjoyed one to two drinks a day. In fact, alcohol can be an excellent social lubricant, and strong social networks are important for maintaining mental and physical health. So, a drink everyday, or now and then, is not bad and can possibly increase your lifespan.

- Eating nuts --- Americans have not always been in love with nuts, but the trend has been changing and it is a good thing. The aisles for nuts in supermarkets and stores are getting bigger and bigger; the market research firms are witnessing increased sales of nuts every year.

A large study in 2021 concluded that people who eat a Mediterranean diet and include a daily portion of nuts have significantly lower risk of heart attacks and strokes. Another recent study published in the New England Journal of Medicine has found that people in the habit of eating a handful of nut, a 4-oz serving, are more likely to live longer compared with people who rarely consume them. The major part of this study in the NEJM was funded by the National Institute of Health. Researchers have shown that a handful of nuts keep you fuller faster, and the sense of satiety helps people eat less, leading to lower risks of diabetes and cardiovascular disease.

Two long-running Harvard studies have linked eating nuts to healthier, longer life. The researchers involved nearly 120,000 participants, beginning in 1980s with a 30-year of follow-up.

There are different kinds of delicious nuts for your choice, but my favorite ones are the walnuts. Walnuts are a great source of omega-3s, protein, polyphenols and vitamin E, fiber, folate, potassium and magnesium. The omega-3 fatty acids, more specifically, the polyunsaturated fatty acids including alpha-linolenic acid (ALA), an anti-inflammatory superstar, can improve skin health, decrease risk of cardiovascular disease and lower the levels of triglycerides. The protein in walnuts helps to support collagen production in the skin, and to prevent age-related muscle loss.

Walnuts also contain polyphenols, phytochemicals with powerful antioxidant and anti-inflammatory properties; they are known to boost your immune system and fight infections. Polyphenols are potent antioxidants which can keep the free radicals in check. Free radicals are unstable molecules that, in excess, can trigger cell damage under oxidative stress, which, over time, can snowball into chronic conditions such as heart disease, diabetes, neurodegenerative disorders and cancer. A report from "Oxidative Medicine and Cellular Longevity "reveals that polyphenols can offer protection against cancer, diabetes and cardiovascular diseases. The studies by the Harvard TH Chan School of Public Health further support that polyphenols are powerful disease fighters, helping to reduce and remove free radicals, protecting the cells from damager, and ultimately keeping chronic diseases at bay

Here are some of the choices for some ' anti-aging ' nuts: Almonds Brazil nuts, cashews, pistachios, and walnuts (ABCPW). So, enjoy your favorite nutty snacks every day while adding some healthy years to your life, why not?

- **Drinking green tea** --- Green tea is the second most consumed beverage in the world, and its health benefits have been touted for centuries. But, it is only relatively recent that medical and scientific studies have been conducted to see specifically what health benefits green tea can give and the mechanisms behind them.

Scientific investigations into the beneficial effects of green tea mostly look at catechins, a type of polyphenols found in considerable amounts in green tea. These phytochemical compounds are a good source of antioxidants which have been shown to have a range of beneficial properties, such as anti-inflammatory, antibacterial, antiviral, anti-diabetic and antimutagenic.

There are several catechins found in green tea, but the EGCG , Epigallocatechin 3-gallate, forms about 50% of the total polyphenols in green tea and is thought to be the major contributor to the green tea benefits. This polyphenol is also the most studies. Besides the polyphenols, green tea contains other compounds such as caffeine, vitamins and trace elements which may contribute to some of the beneficial effects of green tea, though to a lesser extent.

In a study conducted in China with over 100,000 participants, the researchers found that habitual consumption of green tea (at least three cups a day) is associated with lower mortality rates compared to non-tea drinkers. This study suggested that the antioxidants in green tea help protect against cardiovascular disease and reduce the risk factors such as high blood pressure. The habitual tea drinkers, understandably, also had lower risk of strokes, as well as a 29 percent decreased risk of all-cause death, compared to the non-tea drinkers or occasional tea drinkers.

There are two large studies regarding green tea consumption and longevity:

Green tea and mortality study #1 – also called Ohsaki National Health Insurance Cohort Study, researchers looked at 40,530 Japanese adults and followed them for 11 years. They found that those who drink 5 or more cups of green tea a day are 16% less likely to die from any cause than those who drink less than one cup a day. The regular tea drinkers are also 25% less likely to die from heart disease. The most important finding is that green tea may prolong people's lives through reducing the risk of cardiovascular disease and its risk factors. This study was published in the Journal of the American Medical Association in September of 2006.

Green tea and Mortality Study #2 – also named Prospective Shizuoka Elderly Cohort, it is another large study where the scientists from Okayama University of Japan investigated and analyzed 12,251 participants and tracked them for an average of 5 years. After comparing the green tea intake with health in the individuals, the researchers found a clear, convincing pattern – the more green tea consumed, the lower the risk of death from heart disease. More specifically, those drinking seven cups of green tea daily were 75% less likely to die from heart disease, a very remarkable scientific finding!

Studies have shown that loose-leaf green tea has antioxidant content significantly higher than the common tea bags due to, for one thing, less processing. In general, the loose tea leaves seem to offer more health benefits than most supermarket tea-bag types. The beneficent polyphenols in green tea, EGCG, along with its other nutrients make green tea a much better choice than sodas and other sugary beverages. According to studies conducted at Northwest A and F University in Yangling, China, EGCG can help lower insulin resistance, and improve memory impairment. The insulin seems to function better in the Central Nervous System in the presence of EGCG, suggesting that drinking green tea may have a neuroprotective effect on the brain.

Drinking greet tea for its long-term health benefits, it is important to know about the sources of green tea you are drinking every day. Are the tea plantations or fields away from major highways? The closer to a major highway, the higher the levels of lead present in the tea. It is also important to know the regions where the plants of tea leaves come from. Sometimes, it may not be easy to find the answers; in general, there is not too much of a risk in terms of contaminants. Anyway, tea is an optimal beverage of choice, especially during a time of increased stress and burnout nowadays.

- **Drinking Coffee without sugar or cream**
  --- Coffee beans were first discovered by Ethiopia, an African nation many years ago; coffee has become the most common and prevalent beverage in the U.S. today. Coffee is an excellent source of antioxidants, such as trigonelline among other healthful compounds; antioxidants are known to protect against oxidative stress in the body caused by harmful free radicals.

Many studies have shown that regular coffee drinkers are less likely to die than those who do not drink coffee. Researchers from the University of Cranston in Pennsylvania have found that coffee is a top-ranking winner of antioxidants. Coffee beans also contain many vitamins and minerals, such as riboflavin, pantothenic acid, niacin, thiamine, folic acid, zinc, potassium, manganese and magnesium. Certainly, coffee is the biggest source of antioxidants in the Western diet, out-ranking both fruits and vegetables combined. This must not be misconstrued that coffee has more antioxidants than fruits and vegetables, but rather that coffee intake is so common that it contributes more antioxidants to people's intake of antioxidants on average. In other words, if you don't eat fruits or vegetables, drinking coffee may be one of the largest sources in your diet.

There is a plethora of evidence associating regular, moderate coffee drinking with lower risks of cardiovascular disease including coronary artery disease, congestive heart failure and strokes. However, coffee's effects on arrhythmias and hypertension are either neutral or controversial. In the Nurses' Health Study of 83,000 women, researchers tracked their coffee drinkers for 24 years; they discovered that women, who drank 2 to 3 cups of coffee a day without sugar, decreased their risk of stroke by 19%. Women who did not smoke in the study realized and reported even greater benefits, with a much lower risk of stroke

The results of a large, fairly conclusive study titled "Coffee consumption and all-cause and cause-specific mortality " were published in the ' European Journal of Epidemiology '. It analyzed the benefits of drinking coffee by looking at 40 studies that included 3,852,651 participants. The researchers found that regular coffee consumption decreased death rates, irrespective of age, overweight status, alcohol drinking, smoking habit and caffeine content of coffee. Between 2 to 4 cups of coffee per day seem to be of optimum health benefits; 6 or more cups a day are harmful to the heart due to elevated blood pressure., according to an Australian study in 2019 published in the American Journal of Clinical Nutrition.

Several recent studies have shown that coffee drinking can improve cognitive function such as alertness and focusing for Alzheimer's patients. One study published in the European Journal of Neurology found a link between caffeine in coffee and protection against denervation of the brain in the early stages of Alzheimer's disease.

A Harvard study published on November 16, 2015 by Circulation found that moderate coffee drinking is associated with a lower risk of an early death from type-2 diabetes, cardiovascular disease and neurodegenerative disorders such as Parkinson's disease. They suggest that moderate coffee drinking is linked to longevity. Researchers revealed and analyzed data from a total of more than 208,000 men and women over a period of 30 years. The beneficial effects could be due to certain compounds in coffee, such as chlorogenic acid which helps reduce insulin resistance and inflammation.

Medical researchers are finding all kinds of reasons to recommend that cup of joe, primarily because of its content of bioactive compounds, antioxidants-rich polyphenols that promote health and reduce oxidative stress. Studies published in the New England Journal of Medicine show that these compounds can help improve the gut microbiome, aiding digestion and boosting immunity. A large review of studies published in Nutrition Reviews found that your risk of developing type 2 diabetes drops by 6 percent for each cup of coffee you drink per day. This health benefit of coffee is also supported by a study published in the Journal of Internal Medicine.

The health benefits of drinking coffee in moderation are undeniable, and more and more researches have demonstrated the synergistic effects of consuming both coffee and green tea. One study published in November 2021 in PLOS Medicine found that people who drank 2 to 3 cups of coffee and 2 to 3 cups of green tea per day had 30% decrease in incidence of stroke and 28% lower risk for dementia versus those who did not. Among those participants who experienced a stroke during the follow-up period, drinking 2 to 3 cups of coffee a day was associated with 20% lower risk for post-stroke dementia, and those who drank both coffee and tea, the risk for post-stroke dementia was lowered by 50 percent.

Each ' Blue Zone ' undoubtedly has its own unique cultural customs, traditions, and environmental influences, the five zones share a few characteristics in common. One of the commonalities is regular consumption of coffee, particularly Sardinia, Nicoya, and Ikaria. So, enjoy your longevity with your coffee!

The American College of Cardiology at the 2022 scientific seminars, releasing the results of its three-part study with data collected from over 500,000 people who were followed over a 10-year period, have shown that coffee consumption in moderation may lower risk of heart disease and increase life longevity. People who drink 2-3 cups of coffee a day are less likely to have a stroke or dementia. If you already drink 2 to 3 cups of coffee a day, you can continue to do so without fear; however, you should also take your preferences and health history into consideration.

Vitamin C:

It is such a famous micro-nutrient with believers and some skeptics for its multiple health benefits. It is also known as L-ascorbic acid, naturally present in some foods such as citrus fruits, peppers, tomatoes, leafy green vegetables potatoes, Brussels sprouts and strawberries. Vitamin C is not synthesized by the human bodies, and some people prefer taking it in supplement form. Vitamin C is a water-soluble, essential micro-nutrient, important for healthy aging.

Vitamin C is an integral part of many structures of our body, and the body cannot make collagen without vitamin C working as a co-factor. The body actually would fall apart with the protein collagen. The collagen fibers are the most important structural and shock-absorbing component of the connective tissues. Collagen fibers twist around each other to form the scaffolding for the bones, cartilages, skin and muscles. Collagen is also the supportive component of ligament, tendons and blood vessels. Furthermore, collagen keeps your skin from getting wrinkles; you need collagen to grow new skin and form scar tissue when you get a cut.

In fact, vitamin C is necessary to make certain key hormones which include serotonin, dopamine, epinephrine and norepinephrine. Most people who eat a variety of fruits and vegetables daily should have enough of this vitamin from their foods with a healthy lifestyle. However, smokers are found to have lower blood levels of vitamin C than non-smokers because of the considerable amounts of harmful free radicals generated by cigarette smoking. The safe range of vitamin C intake seems to be broad and somewhat controversial, as opposed to the daily recommended guidelines by the U.S. Government.

The optimal physiological amounts and levels vary among different individuals, depending upon one's lifestyle and health status.

Indiscriminate and excessive use of vitamin C can be hazardous, leading to increased secretion of urinary oxalate and uric acid, resulting in the formation of kidney stones. Another potentially dangerous condition, hemochromatosis, due to overload of iron in the body (vitamin C promotes the absorption of iron from the intestines). Excessive supplementation of vitamin C at massive doses may counteract the effect of anti-clotting medications. In general, doses approaching 6 to 8 grams a day can be expected to be unsafe. If you are, like many others, a strong believer in and regular user of vitamin C supplement, it is prudent and advisable to consult your physician.

Tom Kirkwood, an eminent researcher on aging at the University of Newcastle gave a vivid depiction of the biochemical action of vitamin C in 2001:

" When a molecule of vitamin C encounters a free radical, it becomes oxidized and thereby renders the free radical innocuous. The oxidized vitamin C molecule then gets restored to its non-oxidized state by an enzyme called vitamin C reductase. " As we know, some molecules of vitamin C are irretrievably degraded and must be replaced, either by dietary intake or supplements.

Researchers at Cambridge in 2001 reported in the Lancet that the risk of death from any cause was higher in people with low plasma levels of vitamin C, and conversely, that people with high plasma levels of vitamin C were less likely to die within the period studied.

The studies seem to suggest and imply that vitamin C may lengthen lifespan, and this linkage is mainly with dietary intake from fresh, canned or frozen sources.

Paul Linus, a twice Nobel laureate and distinguished Scottish oncologist, Evan Cameron, reported that mega-doses of vitamin C given intravenously could quadruple the survival time of patients with advanced cancer, even bringing complete remission in some cases in their research. As a matter of fact, there is an abundance of research supporting that vitamin C can help keep cancer at bay, according to the U.S. National Institute of Health NIH). The NIH also offers compelling evidence that vitamin C may help prevent age-related macular degeneration and cataract, the two leading causes of vision loss in older people. Vitamin C can help improve heart health, according to a large study involving over 85,000 women; the researchers in the study found that sufficient intake of vitamin C in both dietary and supplemental forms could reduce the risk of coronary artery disease.

Scurvy is no longer a familiar sight, but once a scourge, devastating the lives of sailors, who were deprived of fresh foods including vegetables on their long voyages. These afflicted individuals suffered weakened limbs which became discolored and swollen while their gums bled profusely. Other symptoms of scurvy, which is due to vitamin C deficiency and is rare nowadays, include easy bruising, anemia, fatigue, heart failure and eventually death.

Without adequate supply of vitamin C, one cannot absorb enough iron to stock the red blood cells with hemoglobin, leading to anemia. Many antioxidants require ' partners ' in order to work effectively, and some of these biochemical partners include vitamin C, vitamin E, selenium and co-Q10.

Vitamin C, a powerful antioxidant, is known as an immunity-booster, and can help shorten the duration of a common cold. The U.S. recommended daily allowance (RDA) for an average normal adult is about 100mg; this value can certainly vary when special needs of one's body and health status is considered. There is no question that accumulation of un-neutralized, superfluous free radicals produced in the body are associated with aging and development of chronic diseases, and their harmful attacks on the cells, cellular constituents like DNA and connective tissues are well documented.

Vitamin C is also important for skin health; it stimulates collagen production and may guard against wrinkle development and premature aging of skin due to sun exposure. It may surprise you that vitamin C can help improve your mood because it is essential for the production of neurotransmitters in the brain, dopamine in particular. Dopamine is the ' happy ' neurotransmitter linked to making us feel positive and energized; dopamine plays a vital role in the brain's pleasure and reward systems. Of course, there are a lot of factors that can affect one's mood, vitamin C is just one of them.

Vitamin D:

Vitamin is important for good health, especially in the elderly population. Vitamin D's role in various medical conditions has been the subject of much interest and ongoing research. Vitamin D has been linked to many health benefits from better heart health and bone strength to a stronger immune system. Many researchers have found yet another reason for us to have adequate intake of this micronutrient: cognitive functioning. At least, one in four U.S. adults and one in five UK adults have low levels of this fat-soluble vitamin, and this number goes up during winter and spring in the northern hemisphere when people are typically exposed to less sunlight, the main source of vitamin D. That is why it is also known as the " sunshine vitamin ". Our body can make vitamin D when direct sunlight converts a chemical in the skin into an active form, calciferol.

North of the northern hemisphere during winter and spring, with latitudinal lines connecting San Francisco to Philadelphia or Athens to Beijing, the sun's rays here are just not strong enough, and it is almost impossible for most people to satisfy their vitamin D needs through diet alone, especially the older adults. According to the Harvard School of Public Health, there are at least one billion people worldwide not getting enough vitamin D. A three-pronged approach is indeed necessary to achieve optimal vitamin D levels: sun exposure, foods and supplements. There are two forms of vitamin D:

D2 and D3. D3 (cholecalciferol) is the form of vitamin D actively made and used by the body. Besides the inadequate exposure to the sun, your skin and tissues that are responsible for production of vitamin D might not work as well with the aging process.

Vitamin D is such an important, vital nutrient crucial for your overall well-being. Undoubtedly, vitamin D, the ever-popular vitamin, helps the body functions in multiple ways with many health benefits. Though the health benefits are linked to sufficient and therapeutic high levels of vitamin D, the links do not necessarily prove cause and effect; there can be many other explanations for the associations observed. Let us look at some of those health benefits that vitamin D may play a role:

- Vitamin D assists the body in absorbing calcium alongside phosphorus to help keep your bones, muscles, and teeth in good shape. It also prevents bone weakness, which can lead to falls and fractures. About 30% of phosphate absorption in the gut depends on vitamin D, and phosphate is essential for muscle contraction.
- Several studies have shown that vitamin D can help with brain function by strengthening neural circuits. In a recent study in JAMA Neurology, which measured vitamin D and cognitive function each year in an ethnically diverse group of elderly patients (about half of whom had some form of cognitive impairment at the start of the study), lower levels of vitamin D were associated with accelerated cognitive decline. According to the VITAL study at Harvard University, older people with vitamin D deficiency performed poorly on tests of memory, attention and reasoning compared to people with adequate levels of vitamin D in their blood. Low levels of this vitamin have been found in patients living with Alzheimer's disease, multiple sclerosis and Parkinson's disease. It is currently inconclusive or unclear whether or not vitamin D can help treat or prevent these neurodegenerative disorders, but,

what do you have to lose if you are suffering from these incurable illnesses?

- Female college students who had low levels of vitamin D were more likely to have clinically significant symptoms of depression, according to a 2015 study published in Psychiatry Research. A large meta-analysis of more than 31,000 research participants, published in the British Journal of Psychiatry, found such correlation as well. So, correcting the deficiency of vitamin D can make elderly people happier; this does not necessarily mean that vitamin D deficiency causes depression, but it is clear that vitamin D supports brain health in general.
- Vitamin D deficiency and heart disease are known to go hand in hand. Many studies have shown that subjects with very low levels of vitamin D were about three times as likely to die of heart failure and five times as likely to die of sudden cardiac death. Researchers in a 2019 study suggested that adequate levels of vitamin could help treat hypertension.
- Vitamin D, according to many studies, seems to have some positive impact and benefits on some types of cancer. A 2011 meta-analysis that included more than one million participants found that higher vitamin D intake and higher levels of vitamin D were linked to lower risk of colorectal cancer. Some studies have suggested that there may be a link between higher levels of vitamin D and a lowered risk of breast cancer, especially post-menopausal women. People with higher levels of vitamin D were 35 percent less likely to develop pancreatic cancer than those with lower levels, according to a 20-year study of 120,000 people conducted by researchers from Brigham and Women's Hospital in Massachusetts.

Some studies postulate that low levels of vitamin D may be associated with a higher risk of developing prostate cancer. A small pilot study from the Medical University of South

Carolina in Charleston found that when patients with prostate cancers received 4,000 IU of vitamin D for 60 days, 60% of them showed improvement in their tumors.

- A lack of vitamin D can affect the immune system, leading to increased risk of catching infections, such as COVID-19. In fact, COVID-19 patients with low plasma levels of vitamin D have been shown to have higher risk for hospitalization. Low vitamin D levels are an independent risk factor for having symptomatic COVID-19 with respiratory distress that requires ICU admission and results in increased mortality. A new study out of Israel suggests that having sufficient levels of vitamin D may significantly reduce the chance of becoming seriously ill from COVID-19.

According to the guidelines from the Endocrine Society, older adults 70 years and over should have a dietary intake of 800 IU of vitamin D every day. Most studies have revealed that vitamin D deficiencies among the geriatric population are common, and supervised or careful and judicious supplementation is necessary. Common foods that can provide you with dietary vitamin D include but not limited to:

- Fatty fish, such as sardines, salmon and tuna
- Egg yolks
- Beef liver
- Meats (Beef and pork)
- Cod liver oil
- Mushrooms
- Dried prunes
- Fortified cereals and milk
- Tofu
- Oatmeal

Vitamin E:

Vitamin E has been getting a lot of attention and popularity like its counterpart, vitamin D. This fat-soluble nutrient can be found in many foods including avocado, fruits, vegetables (Spinach and broccoli), cereals, meats, poultry, eggs, olive oil, almonds, peanuts and wheat germ oil. The National Institute of Health states that vitamin E acts as an antioxidant, helping to protect cells from the damage caused by free radicals. Many experts have agreed that vitamin E is a strong defender of the cell membrane because it plays an important role in protecting lipids, the major component of cell membranes, from oxidation.

Neurons are built mostly out of cholesterol and polyunsaturated fatty acids, which are highly susceptible to oxidative damage. Vitamin E, as a potent antioxidant, protects these compounds from oxidation. Patients with Alzheimer's disease have been found to have lower levels of vitamin E in the cerebrospinal fluid that protects and nourishes the brain and spinal cord. Since elevated levels of oxidative stress in the brain may contribute to the development of Alzheimer's disease, and vitamin E may protect the neurons from undergoing oxidative damage, according to some studies. Even though the AD patients in the studies showed mixed results with vitamin E supplementation, bulk of the findings support a beneficial role.

When vitamin E donates electrons directly to the free radicals, rendering them innocuous and harmless. With the neutralization of the free radicals, vitamin E becomes a weakly reactive free radical product, called alpha-tocopheryl, which is then re-converted into stable vitamin E molecules again by accepting electrons from vitamin C. The more the vitamin C available, the quicker the re=generation of vitamin E for antioxidant activities. The chemically reactive free radicals, if unchecked, can initiate a rapid destructive chain reaction, resulting in:

- Cell membrane lipid damage from lipid peroxidation
- Cellular protein damage
- Intracellular DNA damage

- Oxidation of LDL-cholesterol
- Inflammation

Antioxidants, like vitamin E, can stop and modify this destructive chain reaction, neutralizing the free radicals and protecting the body, the brain and heart in particular, from oxidative stress. Let us look at some of the health benefits of vitamin E for the older adults:

- It can help prevent clogging of the arteries that contribute to cardiovascular disease such as atherosclerosis. Studies have shown that patients with atherosclerosis who took vitamin E supplement showed significantly less plaque buildup in the arteries than those in a control group who were taking a placebo. However, one must be careful and judicious about its supplementation because vitamin E supplement can augment the effects of anti-coagulation medications because at high doses, vitamin E can inhibit the aggregation of platelets, and block the clotting activity of vitamin K.
- Vitamin E may improve cognitive performances in patients with Alzheimer's disease, and in conjunction with vitamin C, may slow the development of the disease according to some studies.
- Some recent studies have shown that vitamin E can help control blood sugar and cholesterol levels in people type-2 diabetes, and decrease cardiovascular complications. Researchers discover that up to 40% of diabetic patients have a gene variant (haptoglobin 2-2 gene) that increases oxidative stress and at least doubles the risk of cardiovascular disease. Israel researchers found that when these patients were given vitamin E 400 IU as supplement daily, their risk of cardiovascular events such as stroke and heart attack fell by 50%.
- Vitamin E has enjoyed a reputation for skin health, preventing the effects of aging on skin. As a powerful antioxidant, it is often used to treat scars, acne, and wrinkles

because it promotes cell regeneration of the skin. It can also reduce the sensitivity to the sun in photo-dermatitis; vitamin E can be used to protect against sunburn.
- Some studies have shown that vitamin E may reduce the risk of death from stroke in post-menopausal women.
- Vitamin E is a powerful antioxidant, and can help fight oxidative stress and inflammation by preventing the formation of new free radicals and by neutralizing existing free radicals that would otherwise cause cellular damage.

Vitamin E from foods is generally safe to consume; toxicity usually comes from supplements. The Office of Supplements suggests that the maximum safe daily intake for most adults is 1,000mg of vitamin E per day. People who use vitamin E supplement regularly should keep their daily dosages low and exercise caution. When in doubt, it is important and prudent to consult with your physician and/or nutritionist to avoid any potential adverse side effects of vitamin E. While a vitamin E deficiency is rare in healthy adults, you can be lacking vitamin E due to poor diet or an underlying medical condition such as Crohn's disease or cystic fibrosis, or cigarette smokers.

Here are a few common foods which are good sources of dietary vitamin E:

- Almonds, hazelnuts and peanuts
- Avocado and Kiwi
- Spinach and broccoli
- Shrimp and fish
- Eggs
- Olive oil
- Sunflower seeds

Vitamin B-12:

Vitamin B12 is a water-soluble vitamin that is required for formation of red blood cells, DNA synthesis, and maintenance of normal neurological function. Since it is water-soluble, the body flushes out and eliminates any excess that is not used, so it is unlikely that you can consume too much of it. About 10 to 15 percent of adults, based on conservative estimates, have B-12 deficiency; it is more common in older people. Since many symptoms of its deficiency are similar to quite a few other conditions associated with aging, it is sometimes overlooked. Vitamin B12 is primarily found in animal products, vegetarians of people following a vegan and vegetarian diet can be at risk for B-12 deficiency. One good source of B-12 for pure vegetarians is nutritional yeast, which packs an impressive amount of B-12, over 10 micrograms from half a cup.

Most often a deficiency occurs when the body absorbs the nutrient poorly or none at all due to various conditions such as aging, celiac disease, Crohn's disease, or prolonged use of antacids, over-the-counter acid blockers, or prescription medications used to treat heartburn, gastroesophageal reflux and peptic ulcer disease. Gastric acid in the stomach is needed for B-12 to detach itself from its original protein moiety so it can be absorbed into the blood stream. When you are over 50 years of age, your body normally produces less gastric acid, making older people prone to B-12 deficiency. Heavy drinking can cause gastritis or irritation of stomach lining, and this can lead low levels of stomach acid, resulting in decreased B-12 absorption

B-12 is linked to pernicious anemia. When the stomach does not produce enough of the intrinsic factor, a protein which helps intestine absorb B-12. In pernicious anemia, the body produces large, immature red blood cells that can't carry oxygen throughout the body; thus, leading to weakness, fatigue, pale and yellowish skin without that healthy glow. It is known that intrinsic factor is needed for the intestines to absorb B-12; however, studies have shown that if B-12 supplementation is high enough and B-12 gets absorbed by a passive mechanism anyway when its stomach concentration is high enough.

Vitamin B12 is indeed a powerhouse, and is crucial for a healthy brain and immune system. In fact, its deficiency can cause memory loss, disorientation, difficulty thinking and reasoning, and thus can be mistaken for dementia. Experts advise that people with unexplained cognitive decline should be tested for B-12 deficiency since B-12 works closely with the metabolic processes in the brain. Researchers from Rush University Medical Center in Chicago have shown that participants with low blood levels of vitamin B12 performed poorly on cognitive tests and their brain scan revealed smaller brain volumes. Low B-12 level is an important risk factor for loss of brain volume among older people, and the serum B12 status may be an early marker of brain atrophy, according to neuroscientific research.

Vitamin B12 is crucial for the making for myelin of the central nervous system (the brain and spinal cord). A deficiency of B-12 can cause your hands feeling numb and tingling, a pin-and-needle sensation.

Many studies have shown that getting enough of this vitamin can help reduce the risk for certain types of cancer. One study in the International Journal of Cancer found that those with low vitamin B12 intakes had increased risk for gastric cancer, especially if they smoked. Another study published in Public Health Nutrition found that participants who had higher vitamin B12 intake had a lower risk of colorectal cancer. Even though cause-and-effect relationships cannot be established conclusively in those studies supporting the health benefits of vitamin B12, it is incontrovertibly one of the most important vitamins to consume enough of in order to promote a healthy metabolism and optimal brain function.

Vitamin A:

Vitamin A is a family of essential fat-soluble dietary compounds that contain a retinyl group. This group of important organic compounds include retinol, retinal, retinoic acid and several provitamin A carotenoids, most notably beta-carotene. Due to the perceived potential risk of hypervitaminosis A, pro-vitamin A carotenoids are recommended as the preferred source of this nutrient. However, eating a lot of pro-vitamin A in its plant-form from a diet doesn't carry the same risk, as its conversion to the active form in the body is regulated, and does not build up to toxic levels. If the body does not need to utilize the beta-carotene from the diet to make vitamin A, the beta-carotene, an antioxidant, that remains will circulate in the body to help keep cells healthy.

Beta-carotene belongs to a group of colored pigments called carotenoids, found in many fruits and vegetables. As a precursor to vitamin A, carotenoids give plants such as carrots, sweat potatoes, and apricots their reddish-violet colors. Beta-carotene is converted to retinol, an active form of vitamin A, which is essential for preserving the eyesight. The early symptoms of vitamin A deficiency is night blindness because vitamin A is a major component of the pigment rhodopsin. Rhodopsin is found in the retina of the eyes and extremely sensitive to light. People with vitamin A deficiency can still see normally during the day, but have reduced vision in darkness and at night as their eyes struggle to pick up light at lower levels.

In addition to preventing night-blindness, having adequate intake of beta-carotene can help slow the decline of eyesight in older adults, according to some studies. Age-related macular degeneration (AMD) is the leading cause of blindness in the developed nations. The Age-Related Eye Disease Study found that giving people over the ago of 50 an antioxidant supplement (including beta-carotene) reduced the risk of developing advanced macular degeneration by 25%.

Vitamin A plays an important role in the growth and development of human cells, and its influence on cancer risk due to uncontrolled growth of abnormal cells and its role in cancer prevention is of much interest to medical scientists. In some observational studies, eating higher amounts of vitamin A in the form of beta-carotene has been linked to a decreased risk of certain types of cancer, including Hodgkin's lymphoma, as well as cervical, lung and bladder cancers. At this time, however, the relationship between vitamin A levels in the body and cancer risk is still not fully understood.

Having sufficient vitamin A in your diet helps keep your immune system healthy and function at its best because vitamin A plays a vital role in maintaining your body's natural defenses. It is also involved in the production and function of white blood cells, which help capture and clear bacteria and other pathogens from the bloodstream. Thus, a deficiency of vitamin A can increase your susceptibility to infections and delay your recovery from the illness.

It has been suggested that vitamin A deficiency may increase your risk of developing acne, as it causes an overproduction of the protein keratin in the hair follicles. Acne is a chronic, inflammatory skin disorder, and the exact role that vitamin A plays in its development and treatment remain relatively unclear at this moment.

Vitamin A deficiency is relatively rare in industrialized countries, but fairly common in developing nations, where it is the leading cause of preventable blindness in children, according to the World Health Organization. The National Institute of Health (NIH) recommended male adults to have a daily intake of 3,000 IU of beta-carotene daily, and female adults with an intake of 2,300 IU of beta-carotene daily.

Dementias

First and foremost, let us clarify some of the myths about dementia.

1. Dementia is inevitable with age. This is false because dementia is not a normal part of aging, but the risk does increase with age. In the U.S., if you are aged

   Between 65 and 74, up to 5% risk
   Between 75 and 84, up to 15% risk
   Between 85 and older, your risk is up to 30%

2. Dementia and Alzheimer's disease are the same. This is not quite correct. Alzheimer's disease is a neurodegenerative disorder accounting for 65 to 75% of all dementia cases; it is thus the most common type of dementia. Other types include vascular dementia, Lewis Body dementia, Frontotemporal dementia, mixed dementia and a few others.
3. If a family member has dementia, I am going to get it too. This is not true because majority of dementia cases do not have a strong genetic link and most of the dementia cases are not hereditary.
4. Since age is a risk factor for the development of dementia, it only affects older adults. This is not exactly true because it can affect younger adults in rare cases.
5. The diagnosis of dementia is often misconstrued as the beginning of the end of a normal life. This is false because many individuals with the diagnosis are able to lead active, meaningful and fulfilling lives for a long time with positive impact form the modifiable factors and preemptive

measures. In other words, many people with the diagnosis of dementia can live a normal life.
6. Memory loss always signifies dementia. This is false because we all forget things occasionally. However, memory impairment can be an early symptom of dementia, like Alzheimer's. The point is memory loss does not necessarily signify the start of dementia.

What is dementia?

Dementia is a frightening word; we seem to be hearing about it more and more nowadays, but with much query and misunderstanding by the public. Many surveys show that half of the middle-aged adults worry about getting dementia and the fear of cognitive decline is widespread. In fact, researchers have found that people are more scared of dementia than of other leading causes of death, such as heart disease and stroke. For the sufferers of dementia, there is indeed a never-ending stigma surrounding the illness that isn't present with other illnesses. People are quite open with other illnesses or diagnoses, e.g. ' I have got cancer '. But when it comes to dementia, people are less open about their illness or diagnosis. I think people have accepted it is a part of aging, but it is not. It is caused by diseases.

Our mind is a very ' precious thing '.but it can also be a very ' feeble thing '. According to the National Institute on Aging, dementia is the gradual loss of cognitive functioning – thinking, remembering, and reasoning - to such an extent that it interferes with a person's daily life and activities. Dementia is essentially a group of symptoms and a clinical manifestation of years of neuropathology.

By 2050, the number of Americans living with dementia is expected to reach about 15 million. Among the public health concerns in the U.S., it is one of the top seven. In general, dementia is characterized by the following impairments:

- Impairment of cognitive ability including language
- Impairment of memory, short term and/or long term

- Impairment of social functioning and the ability to perform activities of daily living (ADL), usually in later stages.

Dementia is a term used to describe a group of symptoms affecting the memory, thinking, reasoning and social abilities severely enough to interfere with one's daily life. Dementia is not a specific disease, and quite a few health conditions can cause dementia. Depending on the cause, some dementia symptoms may be reversible. Symptoms of dementia as defined by the Diagnostic and Statistical Manual of Mental Disorders IV (DSM-IV) include:

- Memory loss
- Aphasia- language problems, loss of vocabulary
- Apraxia- difficulty directing arm and leg movements
- Agnosia- inability to recognize familiar faces and objects
- Impaired visual perception
- Impaired executive functioning, decision making
- Withdrawal from social behaviors

The mere mention of dementia can spark anxiety and fear in anyone who is aging and experiencing cognitive decline. These concerns, unfortunately often ripple into the psyche of family members, close friends and loved ones. Part of the challenge is the many unknowns and uncertainties that accompany dementia. Though there is currently no cure for dementia, many, if not most, inflicted with this ' curse ', live for many years or even decades as the syndrome progresses gradually on a case-by-case basis.

There are different clinical tools to assess one's mental health, but to detect whether someone is having a cognitive problem, the information and description from a family member, a spouse or significant other, or a close friend is more reliable than the person's opinion of their memory and thinking skills. During the initial medical examination, questionnaires for measuring cognitive impairment should be completed by someone who knows the patient well. It is important to know how well does the patient function in the real world.

Dementia per se can be caused by different diseases and conditions, while Alzheimer's disease account for about 70 to 75 percent of all cases. Other neurodegenerative disorders with a dementia component include Parkinson's disease, Huntington's disease and multiple sclerosis. Some psychiatric disorders like depression and schizophrenia can have a component of dementia. Certain infections can cause dementia such as syphilis, meningitis and encephalitis. Although dementias share certain characteristics, each type has a distinct underlying pathology.

There are five behavioral changes as early indicators of dementia, in general:

- Apathy – a decline in interest, motivation and drive,
- Affective dysregulation – Anxiety or worrying about simple and routine things. Mood instability or unexplained sadness
- Lack of impulse control – inability to delay gratification, e.g. shoplifting is not uncommon, and a propensity to get into gambling.
- Social inappropriateness – such as talking to strangers surprisingly, or saying rude or odd things.
- Abnormal perception or thoughts – suspicious of other people's intention or think that other people are planning to harm them or steal their belongings.

Alzheimer's disease:

It is the most common type of dementia, accounting for about 70 to 75% of all dementia cases. Currently in the U.S., there are about six million Americans suffering from Alzheimer's disease, and it is the fifth leading cause of death for adults in the U.S. aged 65 or older, according to the Center for Disease Control and Prevention (CDC). It is a sad, neurodegenerative disorder with multiple dimensions and causalities. Memory impairment and loss tend to be an early sign of Alzheimer's disease, but usually not the case of other types of dementia. Alzheimer's can start years before noticeable signs and symptoms. The American Academy of Neurology estimates that the number of Americans affected by Alzheimer's disease will triple by 2050

It is a heart-breaking disease in which the dearest-loved ones can turn into strangers. But I would like to emphasize that Alzheimer's disease is not a normal part of aging, even though people who live to 85 or older may have up to 50% chance to have this terrible disease. Statistically, it is more common in women than men. The signs and symptoms are numerous and can be subtle, some of them may not be readily apparent to family members, close friends or caregivers. Its signs and symptoms can get worse as the day goes on, called 'sun downing '. They can continue through the night, often resulting in sleep disorders.

In 1906, Dr. Alois Alzheimer in Frankfurt, Germany, was curious about one of his patients, named Auguste D, who lost her memories and did not know the names and use of certain family objects. His patient was also confused, exhibiting strange behaviors at times such as dragging her bed=sheets around during one of his home visits. He performed an autopsy, and microscopically, he found sticky deposits around the neurons which later researchers called amyloid plaques. Some tangles of tau protein were also found inside the neurons intracellularly in the brains of some Alzheimer's patients. At the time, Dr. Alois Alzheimer in 1907 gave the diagnosis of presenile dementia, which was later named after him, the Alzheimer's disease.

Today, beta amyloid plaques and fibrillary Tau tangles are the two most important pathological, cellular features of the disease. However, tangles can occur in the absence of the amyloid plaques; nevertheless, the presence of beta-amyloid plaques and neuro-fibrillary tangles serve to increase the risk for development of Alzheimer's disease. Interestingly, some older people seem relatively resistant to the development of the disease as researchers have discovered, despite an abundance of plaques and tangles in the brain confirmed by imaging. Their cerebral functions are incredibly preserved even at advanced age. They are able to live without mental frailty and cognitive dysfunction. Thus, it is possible to resist and overcome the genetic and pathological forces, and indeed Alzheimer's disease is not an inevitable consequence of aging!

Measurable and subjective signs and symptoms of Alzheimer's disease usually appear years before a diagnosis is made; they are subtle, but fairly obvious at times. Family and friends, without being attentive and suspecting, often disregard those signs and symptoms as parts of getting old. In fact, misdiagnoses of patients with Alzheimer's are not uncommon, especially in the early stage of this disorder. Memory problems are typically the first signs of cognitive impairment in Alzheimer's. Some forgetfulness is normal with aging, but certain types of memory problems can be a red flag for Alzheimer's, such as:

- Forgetting recently learned information or events
- Forgetting important dates, like Thanksgiving Day or spouses' birthdays
- Forgetting where you have placed certain items, like car keys or a cell phone, and being unable to retrace steps to find them
- Asking the same questions again and again
- Trouble with familiar tasks
- Getting lost in familiar places like in own neighborhood, or on a frequently traveled route

Sometimes, the individuals with Alzheimer's can act like a child and become dependent completely on a certain member of the family and constantly follow them around as shadowing. One of the earliest changes in judgment for Alzheimer's patients is the handling of money, They might give money to unworthy strangers like telemarketers, or withhold money that should be paid such as utility bills. Moreover, Alzheimer's patients will have difficulty keeping track of the regular monthly bills even though they were able to manage them before.

They might put the car keys in the freezer of the refrigerator; they have a tendency to walk and wander aimlessly. In some cases, he or she might leave the house in the middle of the night to find a toilet for a physical need because they do not realize that they are at home. The affected persons may stop in a discussion or in the middle of a conversation and have no clue how to continue; they simply have trouble following or joining a conversation. They may pass a mirror and think another person is in the room due to visual problem of perception. Alzheimer's patients may have trouble operating familiar household equipment and appliances at home including microwave and washing machine.

Alzheimer's patients may not dress themselves appropriately or groom themselves properly. They can also suffer from visual-spatial relationships, leading to difficulty with balance and judging distance; thus, driving can become problematic and uneasy partly due to disruption of depth perception. Cognitive abilities are damaged unevenly and at different times in the disease process; the Alzheimer's patients will be able to do something but not others. It is possible for the disease to damage one part of the brain without affecting the other as much. The gradual loss of taste is rather subtle, and the affected person may show it as loss of appetite even for their favorite foods.

Nobody really knows or can predict how this dementing illness will unfold. It is such an agonizing, cruel process to see how Alzheimer's disease destroys the mind with mental and physical decline over time. It is likened to watching a tragic, slow motion picture, but not knowing when it is going to end, for better or worse. Of course, this must be very unsettling, heart-breaking, and depressing for the caregiver facing uncertainty every day; I do not doubt that the patient feels the same. Nobody, even the best expert, can figure out what the impaired person understood or intended because our brain is so complex beyond human comprehension.

If you recognize some of the signs and symptoms of Alzheimer's disease in a family member or someone you love and care about, it is important to talk with a healthcare professional. Trust your instinct and ' gut feeling '. Denial is common during the early stages of Alzheimer's. Although there is no cure for Alzheimer's disease at this time, you should seek advice from and work with the healthcare professional who can diagnose the condition and recommend the best ways to manage the symptoms and provide holistic support. On this long journey of pain and suffering, trials and tribulations, as a caregiver, you are traveling together with your loved one with brain impairment. You will need to pray for wisdom, strength and equanimity to endure.

One striking thing I want to share with my readers who are taking care of loved ones diagnosed with Alzheimer's disease, or suspicious of this dementing illness. When my wife survived a major stroke, her brain imaging also confirmed multiple micro-infarcts and the amyloid deposition. Her recovery from the stroke was satisfactory with physical therapy and rehabilitation; but she seems to have lost her smiles along with some of the signs and symptoms highly suggestive of Alzheimer's disease. She does not get excited or take joy in life's simple pleasures such as favorable meal, funny jokes I tell, or hilarious sitcom on television. This inexplicable and profound loss of feeling pleasure can certainly be one of the early signs of Alzheimer's. This lack of, or the unfortunate, impaired ability to experience pleasure, called anhedonia, can be observed by many caregivers of Alzheimer's patients also, and probably caused by degeneration and deterioration of the brain's pleasure center.

Because of their fading abilities in expressing, relating and articulating, caregivers, friends and family often find long silences and pauses during conversations at a gathering. The affected person, while sitting at the dining table eating with family, can lapse into complete silence, staring in the space and absorbed in thought for some time. As the memory and cognitive skills continue to worsen, significant and disturbing personality changes may take place and the patients really require extensive care. Dementia becomes more pronounced and less manageable, making independent living essentially impossible and dangerous. The patients sadly become totally bed-ridden and incontinent. At this time, hospice can be of great benefit to both the caregiver and the patient in the final stage of the disease.

Many patients with Alzheimer's disease can live five to ten years after diagnosis, but some can live as long as 20 years, depending on other factors. Most of the Alzheimer's patients are receiving their care at home from their family, either the spouse, a close relative, or adult children. With the expected increase of Alzheimer's cases, the number of caregivers will also rise considerably with millions of hours of unpaid care with much unspoken personal sacrifice and enormous costs to society. Taking care of your loved one with Alzheimer's at home is a totally uncharted territory and experience for many people. As a devoted caregiver for your loved one suffering from Alzheimer's disease, the challenges can be overwhelming, to say the least.

Keep in mind that the caregiver of Alzheimer's patient is living with many unexpected incidents and/or episodes which may not make any sense at all. These happenings can be very frustrating, irritating, embarrassing and exhausting. Understandably, this can wear you out even the most patient and loving caregiver. Despite the resilience of human beings and the steadfast devotion of the caregiver, our psychological/physiological balance can be pushed over the edge, becoming dysregulated and dysfunctional if it is tax beyond the limits to adapt and respond. Furthermore, the pressures of daily living and coping can reach a point where the caregiver is constantly in a state of hyper-arousal, reacting constantly to the multiple stressors, and eventually leading to the feelings of helplessness and hopelessness.

Researchers in social science have observed that although it may be difficult to admit how they feel, Alzheimer's caregivers often experience, over time and subconsciously, anger or deep=seated resentment towards those they love and care for – I call it 'reactive ambiguity '. The feelings of anger and frustration and hopelessness can conceal your pain, grief, resentment and despair at a deeper level, even though it may not be easy to acknowledge or accept at a conscious level because this is clearly and ironically in conflict with the caregivers' sense of love, devotion and duty. There is no doubt that this conflicting predicament or reactive ambiguity is very likely to adversely impact the caregivers' health with potentially stupendous costs to our society, and this dimension of Alzheimer's disease must be taken seriously.

Vascular dementia:

This type of dementia is also called multi-infarct dementia, accounting for 20 to 25% of dementia cases. The second most frequent type of dementia after Alzheimer's disease. Depending on the areas pf the brain being infarcted or damaged, vascular dementia can have variable signs and symptoms. Some vascular dementias may not get worse, become stabilized and even show improvement with successful rehabilitation, if further strokes can be prevented. When symptoms of both vascular dementia and Alzheimer's co-exist, they are called mixed dementia. But unlike Alzheimer's disease, the most significant symptoms of vascular dementia tend to involve the speed of thinking and problem solving rather than memory loss which can be affected.

Vascular dementia is the result of certain health conditions that damage the brain's blood vessels, and reduce their ability to supply the brain with the amounts of nutrition and oxygen it needs to perform thought processes effectively. These conditions that may lead to vascular dementia include:

- Brain hemorrhage – it is often caused by high blood pressure weakening a blood vessel leading to bleeding into the brain.
- Ischemic stroke – this anatomically blocks an artery of the brain, causing a range of symptoms that may include vascular dementia. Some of these strokes don't cause any noticeable symptoms; however, these silent strokes still increase dementia risk.
- Narrowed and hardening of blood vessels that supply the brain (atherosclerosis).

Therefore, vascular dementia is characterized by an array of symptoms which include:

- Unilateral, focal weakness
- Slowed thinking
- Trouble with speech
- Confusion
- Reduced ability to organize thoughts or actions
- Unsteady gait
- Inability to control urination

- Difficulty paying attention
- Restlessness
- Personality changes
- Some memory impairment

Early signs and symptoms of vascular dementia may include:

- Having difficulty performing familiar tasks
- Getting lost on familiar routes
- Having trouble finding the right words for common and familiar objects
- Misplacing things and unable to trace them
- Changes in personality, behaviors and social skills

When changes in thought processes and reasoning occur rather suddenly after a stroke, and seem clearly linked to a stroke, this condition is called post-stroke dementia. However, vascular dementia in most of the cases, develop gradually, just like Alzheimer's disease, and often occur together. Many studies show that many people with vascular dementia also have Alzheimer's disease.

Physicians performing a neurologic examination may notice subtle or not so subtle signs suggesting there may have been a stroke at some point. This type of progressive neurodegeneration with multiple small tiny strokes accumulating in damaged areas of the brain look like microscopic potholes in brain scans.

The risk factors for the development of vascular dementia are relatively straight-forward and these include:

- Increasing age, usually after 65.
- History of heart attack or stroke
- Atherosclerosis
- High blood sugar levels
- High cholesterol and triglyceride levels
- Cigarette smoking

- Atrial fibrillation, which increases the risk of stroke because it can cause blood clots (thrombi) to form in the heart that can dislodge and go to the blood vessels of the brain.

The single most important differentiator of dementia versus normal aging is what people often call " benign senescent forgetfulness ", which is generally considered to be a normal age-related memory phenomenon. In benign senescent forgetfulness, the ' normal' older person still has the ability to re-learn, if they forget something, As for the people with dementia, they struggle with re-learning what they forget. That is the clinical difference!

Lewy-body dementia:

It may be the third most common type of progressive dementia after Alzheimer's dementia and vascular dementia, with more men affected than women. In the early 1900s, while researching Parkinson's disease, the neuro-scientist Friederich L. Lewy discovered abnormal protein deposits that affect the brain's normal functioning. These abnormal protein deposits of alpha=synuclein are collectively called Lewy bodies. Lewy bodies can be found in the brain stem where they disrupt and deplete the neurotransmitter dopamine, causing Parkinsonian symptoms. Lewy bodies can also be found in the synapses of neurons in the cerebral cortex, causing problems in perception, thinking and behavior due to depletion of acetylcholine. Therefore, with its wide range of symptoms, Lewy body dementia (LBD) can be hard to diagnose because of the symptoms similar to Alzheimer's dementia and Parkinson disease dementia. Unfortunately, Lewy Body Dementia becomes over time, and there is no cure currently. However, Lewy Body Dementia is different from the classic Parkinson's dementia because Lewy Body Dementia comes on at the same time as the movement problems like tremor, stiffness and slowness. With the involvement of the Autonomic Nervous System, LBD can lead to poor regulation of bodily functions such as bowel movements, urinary bladder control, and blood pressure (orthostatic hypotension). Vivid visual hallucinations are particularly common in Lewy Body Dementia, and can start fairly early in the course of the disease.

Like Alzheimer's disease, Lewy Body Dementia can cause memory loss, confusion, impaired concentration, and poor attention. Like Alzheimer's disease, LBD can affect the ability to recognize faces and to judge distances.

Parkinson's Disease:

It is a chronic, progressive neurodegenerative/movement disorder, and a majority of the patients develop dementia; but the time from the onset of movement symptoms to the onset of dementia symptoms varies greatly from patient to patient. Dementia, unfortunately, is a comorbidity of Parkinson's, which means the damage caused by it to the brain can cause dementia. In one study of men at age 70 with Parkinson's disease without dementia, the participants have a life expectancy of 8 years, of which 5 years would be expected to be dementia-free and 3 years would be expected to be with dementia. Thus, dementia is a key, critical part of survival in Parkinson's disease, and must be planned for preemptively for the patients and families. Some of the autopsy studies have revealed that people with Parkinson's disease often have amyloid plaques and tau tangles similar to those found in people with Alzheimer's disease, but the mechanisms are not clearly understood. In one study, at

Parkinson's disease usually occur in people who are 50 or older, and is more common in men than women. The early-onset form of Parkinson's can be seen in people younger than 50. It arises from decreased or depleted dopamine production in the brain, and the absence of dopamine makes it hard for the brain to coordinate muscle movements. The lack of or, low levels of dopamine also contribute to mood and cognitive problems later in the course of the disease.

At the onset, symptoms of Parkinson's disease are usually mild, and then progressively get worse. The first signs and symptoms are often subtle with some tremors in the hands, arms and legs. Walking is stiff and slow with trouble maintaining balance and coordination. Friends and family will notice changes in the affected person's handwriting if they are attentive. As the disease progresses, other symptoms include depressed mood, trouble chewing and swallowing foods, weight loss, hallucination, dementia and others. Parkinson's disease dementia can cause problems with speaking and communications with others, forgetfulness, impaired memory, understanding abstract concepts and inability to pay attention.

There is no cure for Parkinson's disease other than symptomatic treatment, currently. We don't understand clearly or conclusively how or why dementia often occurs with Parkinson's disease. Eventually, the dementia will affect the person's ability to care for themselves. Physical, occupational, and speech therapy can help your ability to care for yourself and communicate with other people, while creating a safe environment such as installing grab bars in the bathroom, removing obstacles like throw area rugs and loose carpets, and keeping frequently used items within reach.

Frontotemporal Dementia (FTD):

This is not a common type of dementia with a strong genetic component, in other words, FTD often runs in the family. It is characterized by the breakdown of neurons and their connections in the frontal and temporal lobes of the brain. This clinical syndrome is associated with atrophy or shrinking of the frontal and temporal anterior lobes of the brain.

Originally known as Pick's disease, the symptoms of Frontotemporal dementia fall into two clinical patterns that involve either (1) changes in behavior, or (2) problems with the language and speech. Currently, there are no treatments available to cure or slow the progression of FTD. FTD tends to occur at a younger age, between the ages of 40 and 65.

Signs and symptoms vary, depending on which part of the brain is affected. Behavioral changes, which can be extreme, include:

- Loss of inhibition
- Loss of interest (apathy)
- Loss of empathy

- Increasingly inappropriate behavior
- Neglect of personal hygiene
- Poor judgment, or none at all
- Repetitive compulsive behaviors or habits
- Abnormal eating behavior, overeating or eating inedible things
- Inappropriate sexual behavior or becoming more sexually demonstrative
- Lack of social tact.

Language and speech problems of FTD include:

- Difficulty in using and understanding written and spoken language due to trouble finding the right word to use in speech or naming objects
- Making errors in sentencing construction
- Not knowing the meanings of words

As the conditions worsen, the impaired individuals may engage in dangerous behaviors or be unable to care for themselves. 24-hour nursing care at home become necessary or full-time nursing home placement is unavoidable.

Huntington's disease:

It is also known as Huntington's chorea, a rare hereditary neurodegenerative disorder affecting a person's cognition and thinking, movements and emotion. It usually occurs between the 40s and 50s; when the condition develops before age 20, it is called juvenile Huntington's disease. The symptoms of the juvenile form are somewhat different and the disease may progress more rapidly.

Huntington's disease is caused by an inherited defect in a single gene. It is an autosomal dominant genetic disorder, which means that a person needs only one copy of the defective gene to develop the disease. From the onset or emergence of the disease to death can range from 10 to 30 years. Eventually, the affected person requires assistance with all activities of daily living and care, and be confined to a bed in the later stages of the disease.

The symptoms of movement problems can be both involuntary and voluntary:

- Rigidity and contracture of muscles (dystonia)
- Involuntary jerking or writhing (twisting and squirming) movements of the body – chorea
- Abnormal eye movements (nystagmus)
- Problems with gait, balance and posture
- Difficulty with speech and/or swallowing

Cognitive symptoms include:

- Difficulty focusing or organizing
- Lack of impulse control
- Difficulty in learning new information
- Slowness in thinking
- Lack of awareness of one's own abilities and behaviors

Psychiatric symptoms are common with major depression as the prominent feature. Others include:

- Feelings of sadness and apathy.
- Social withdrawal
- Loss of energy and fatigue
- Obsession with death or suicide
- Irritability and insomnia
- Bipolar

People with a known family history of Huntington's disease may consider genetic counseling and testing, and family planning options.

Dr. Richard Ng, B.S., D.O.

Creutzfeldt-Jakob Disease (CJD):

It is a rare disorder, usually with a rapid progression of dementia symptoms; it is first described in 1920, with one to two cases per million per year worldwide, according to epidemiological statistics. CJD belongs to a group of rare brain disorders known as ' prion disease ' in which the prion, a glyco-protein misfolded into an abnormal three-dimensional shape. The misshapen infectious prions can disrupt and harm normal biological processes and spread within the brain rather rapidly, thus, CJD is a type of dementia which progresses fast, unlike Alzheimer's, Lewy Body Dementia, or Frontotemporal dementia which typically has a slower progression.

The misfolded prions destroy brain cells, leading to rapid decline in the affected person's thinking and reasoning. Other symptoms include confusion and disorientation, mood changes and vision problems. With impaired functions of muscles, the patient has difficulty walking. This transmissible spongiform encephalopathy is sometimes called the human form of " Mad Cow Disease ".

In acquired CJD, the terrible disease is transmitted by exposure to brain or nervous system tissues, usually through certain surgical procedures. The iatrogenic transmission of CJD agent has been reported; these cases were linked to the use of contaminated human growth hormone, dura mater and corneal grafts, or neurosurgical equipment. All of these equipment-related cases occurred before the routine implementation of sterilization procedures currently used in healthcare facilities. No such cases have been reported since 1976.

Treatable and reversible dementia

Some causes of dementia or dementia-like symptoms are treatable and reversible, with modifiable contributing factors such as:

- Hypoxia and Anoxia – they are fairly common causes of dementia, which is usually short-lived and reversible if corrective measures are quickly and appropriately instituted
- Dehydration – dementia-like symptoms can occur as a result of not drinking enough fluids, more specifically, water. Most of us tend to take water for granted, and ironically, chronic dehydration is quite common. Many people are not aware of , or do not realize the paramount importance of adequate water intake for physical and mental health. The human body is about 70% water, whereas the human brain is at least 75% water and is very sensitive to any degree of dehydration at cellular levels. Water is not just a simple, inert substance; it is life-giving and life-sustaining. Water is critical in the production of electrical energy for all brain functions, including thinking. One of the first signs of dehydration is " brain fog " – being unable to concentrate and having difficulty remembering things. Other mental symptoms of dehydration include: confusion, headache, mental slowness, increased irritability and fatigue.

    As we get older, we lose the sharpness, acuity and precision of our senses, including hearing, vision, thirst, taste and smell. The gradual loss of the sense of thirst makes the elderly more susceptible to dehydration; this phenomenon has profound, detrimental effects on the elderly, both mentally and physically. Studies by Phillips and Associates have shown that after 24 hours of water deprivation, the elderly participants still do not realize that they are thirsty. Other studies published in the Lancet have supported the conclusion that the thirst mechanism is gradually lost in the elderly with aging.

The human body has not any stored water to draw from in case of dehydration; that is why we must drink water regularly and throughout the day. An important scientific paper by Ephraim Katchaski-Katzir of the Weitzmann Institute demonstrated that proteins and enzymes function more effectively in solutions of lower viscosity, i.e. they need adequate water in their immediate milieu to work optimally. The most significant complication and consequences of dehydration is the loss of necessary essential amino acids in the production of neurotransmitters. Therefore, chronic dehydration can disrupt neuronal function and cause neurological damage to the brain because the raw materials become less available for the brain to produce neurotransmitters.

- ## Normal Pressure Hydrocephalus:

The disease was first described by Salomon Hakim and Adams in 1965. The brain has chambers called ventricles that normally contains special clear liquid, called cerebrospinal fluid (CSF). CSF circulates around in the brain and spinal cord, cushioning and protecting the Central Nervous System from damage. Under normal homeostasis, the body just makes enough CSF each day and absorbs that same amount. Sometimes, too much fluid can build up in the ventricles, causing damage to the brain, condition called hydrocephalus, usually normal-pressure (NPH).

This abnormal condition occurs most often in people over age 60, diagnosed by a CT or MRI and spinal tap. Risk factors for NPH include: older age 60 and over, history of head injury, or brain infection, brain tumor and/or brain surgery. There is a triad of symptoms: Difficulty walking or gait disturbance, dementia, and impaired bladder control (urinary incontinence).

The followings are possible symptoms of NPH: abnormal gait and trouble walking, poor balance and prone to falling, confusion with forgetfulness, mood changes with lack of interest in social activities, and loss of control of urinary bladder. A commonly used and relatively successful treatment for NPH is the ' shunt ' procedure: a tube is placed surgically into the brain and inserted into a ventricle to drain the excess fluid. The shunt is then passed underneath the skin from the head through the neck and chest to the abdomen where the body absorbs it. The shunt stays in place as long as there is too much CSF in the brain.

- Hypoglycemia:

    People with hypoglycemia (low blood sugar) can develop dementia-like symptoms or personality changes, through a variety of mechanisms such as damage to the cerebral cortex and/or hippocampus, neuronal dysfunction, loss of ionic homeostasis, increase in the levels of Reactive Oxygen Species (ROS), and augmented production of amyloid precursor proteins.

    Mild to moderate episodes of hypoglycemia usually do not require treatment, but severe episodes often lead to hospitalization due to serious symptoms such as dizziness, confusion, disorientation and even seizures.

In the last two decades, cardiovascular morbidity and mortality have been considerably reduced in people with diabetes mellitus through intensive and aggressive management of multiple risk factors. However, in parallel with and contrary to this trend, the prevalence and clinical significance of neurodegenerative disorders are steadily increasing. Hypoglycemia has become a ' dangerous ' clinical situation in the strict management and treatment pf diabetes; in fact, it is well known as an important factor that directly affects the risk of dementia and cognitive impairment, according to some studies.

Ironically, it is well known that uncontrolled diabetes is associated with an increased risk for Alzheimer's disease and other age-related dementias in the elderly patients. The thinking has been that aggressive treatment to achieve tight glycemic control would lower the risk, but many new studies including Harvard experts, suggest that such approach and treatment may do more harm than good in older patients if their blood sugar drop to very low levels. Recent research that sees and suggests a link between dangerously low blood sugar and dementia in older patients with type-2 diabetes raises more questions about the strategy of aggressively treating diabetic patients to achieve tight glycemic control. Older patients in new studies whose blood sugar fell so low that they ended up in the hospital were found to have a higher risk for dementia than patients with no history of treatment for low blood sugar, medically known as hypoglycemia.

Type-2 diabetes has reached an epidemic proportion nowadays, and most of us agree that we are going to see more dementia than we have ever seen before as these diabetic patients age. A large clinical trial sponsored by the National Heart Lung and Blood Institute reported their findings that aggressive treatment to achieve blood sugar levels similar to those seen in people without diabetes was linked to an increased risk of death in older people with type-2 diabetes. The study clearly raised the safety concerns about the use of aggressive treatment to achieve tight glucose control in older patients. Episodes of hypoglycemia can lead to falls, fractures, seizures, head injuries, and problems with memory and thinking. As a caveat, a blood sugar level that is a little high is less dangerous than a low blood sygar level, especially in older people.

- **Vitamin B-12 deficiency:**

    Vitamin B-12 or cobalamin is important for maintaining healthy neurons and red blood cells. Vitamin B-12 deficiency is common in older adults and vegetarians; it is found naturally in foods that come from animals, including fish, meat and poultry. Some studies suggest that low vitamin B-12 levels may be associated with an increased risk of dementia. Vitamin B-12 supplementation seemed to have improved memory in Alzheimer's patients in some observational studies, but evidences are inconclusive.

    Vitamin B-12 is needed to make red blood cells, and its deficiency can lead to megaloblastic anemia compromising and reducing oxygen supply to tissues and organs. Absorption of vitamin B-12 by the body requires intrinsic factor from the stomach; patients with history of gastric resection are at high risk of cobalamin deficiency.

    There is an increasing evidence that vitamin B-12 deficiency is associated with a variety of hematological, neurological and psychiatric problems. The symptoms include:

    - Pallor of skin
    - Weakness and fatigue

- Paresthesia (sensation of pins and needles), a common complaint among patients with neurologic symptoms
- Oral ulcers
- Glossitis (smooth and tender tongue)
- Dizziness
- Tachycardia
- Feeling breathless, especially with exertion
- Headache
- Mood changes
- Dementia with memory loss

The incidence of low vitamin B-12 levels among dementia patients has been found to range between 29% and 47% in some studies. The electrophysiological signs of demyelination can be detected in tests of nerve conduction velocity and somatosensory evoked potentials in patients with vitamin B-12 deficiency, however, the exact mechanism of myelin damage following B-12 deficiency is still unknown. In a study with patients suffering from vitamin B-12 deficiency after gastric resections, 50% showed intellectual impairments.

Hypovitaminosis is one of the few dementia-causing disorders that are treatable and reversible today, despite skepticism by some. Anyway, all patients with cognitive impairment, or suspicion thereof, should be investigated for vitamin B-12 deficiency.

Depression:

This negative emotion and mental disorder along with its clinical manifestation has reached an epidemic proportion in our stressful, hectic society. Some researchers believe that depression predates the onset of Alzheimer's disease, and constitutes a distinct risk factor. There are many observational studies showing the prevalence of depression among Alzheimer's patients, ranging from 20% to 40%. However, the link between depression and Alzheimer's dementia is not clear: Is depression an emotional response to the terrible loss caused by the illness? Or, depression itself makes the persons more susceptible to the development of dementia? This takes us back to the proverbial question: " which is first, chicken or egg " ?

There is no doubt that depression and dementia are both common conditions in older people, and they, in fact, often occur together. Depression can simulate symptoms of dementia in elderly individuals, resulting is a high rate of misdiagnosis. When depression is mistaken as dementia, the phenomenon is called pseudo-dementia with an apparent intellectual decline due to a lack of energy or effort. People with pseudo-dementia are often forgetful, moving slowly, showing low motivation and mental slowness. This syndrome generally responds well to treatment for depression, and as the mood improves, the person's energy level, ability to concentrate, and intellectual functioning usually return to previous levels. In other words, depressed senior citizens may experience symptoms of confusion, memory problems, difficulty concentrating, and fatigue that are easily treatable with psychiatric care. An important part of the treatment for depression is psychosocial to improve social connections.

Things that can keep depression at bay – socializing with friends and family, pursuing hobbies, and being physically active -- also help mental function sharp. People who are depressed often withdraw from social contact, which can accelerate mental deterioration. Social isolation that is the result of depression can be very detrimental to brain health. Social connection is important for brain stimulation and mental health.

Depression and dementia share certain features, but there are some differences that help distinguish one from the other:

- The decline in mental functioning tends to be more rapid with depression than with Alzheimer's disease
- People with depression are more likely to notice their forgetfulness and comment on their memory troubles, while those suffering from Alzheimer's may seem indifferent to such changes of memory impairment. There is such a phenomenon called depression-related memory loss; when

one is depressed, you are more likely to recall sad memories, feeling like nothing good ever happens. Furthermore, the disassociation from the brain can cause memory loss or brain fog.
- People with depression are usually not disoriented, unlike Alzheimer's patients with visuo-spatial dysfunction
- People with depression have difficulty concentrating in general, whereas Alzheimer's patients simply have problems with memory
- People with depression are able to maintain their writing, speaking and motor skills; this is not the case with Alzheimer's disease after the early stages

Sleeping disorders:

Getting enough sleep is a challenge for many of us nowadays, especially as we age, and there is a plethora of evidence that adequate, quality sleep is crucial for maintaining a healthy brain. Several studies recently have linked " sleep apnea " , a condition in which a person wakes up several times during the night gasping for air, in older people to increased mental impairment. In the U.S., sleep deprivation is common even though most people do not realize it, or simply ignore it , being unaware of the potential adverse and negative impact on our health and general well-being.

Researchers have shown that chronic sleep deprivation causes increased deposition of beta-amyloid plaques in the brain, thus raising the risk for development of Alzheimer's disease, the most common form of dementia. We all need adequate, quality sleep , which allows the brain to rest and reset. This " down time " is crucial and necessary so that neurotoxic and metabolic wastes can be eliminated optimally. Older people are usually light sleepers and they spend less time in the deep stages of the sleep cycle. Getting a restful night's sleep for them is often complicated by some physical ailments with aches and pains. It must be pointed out that during deep sleep, also known as rapid eye movement (REM) sleep, the body including the brain heals and recharges itself.

A recent study has found that older people who are prescribed a device to treat their Obstructive Sleep Apnea (OSA) may have a lower risk of developing Alzheimer's disease and other forms of dementia. Researchers at Michigan Medicine's Sleep Disorders Center looked at 53,321 Medicare recipients over age 65 who had been diagnosed with OSA. This retrospective study by the medical scientists noted that people who used positive airway pressure devices (commonly known as CPAP) as prescribed were less likely to be diagnosed with dementia or Alzheimer's disease in the next three years than people who did not use CPAP. The findings of the study clearly showed that positive airway pressure (PAP) therapy was associated with lower odds for a diagnosis of incident Alzheimer's disease and also lower odds of mild cognitive impairment (MCI).

There is no doubt that chronic sleep deprivation or sleep disruption is bad for mental health. Recent research, which followed about 8,000 people in their early 50s for a period of 25 years ; those participants who slept less than six hours a night are 30% more likely to develop dementia later on in life usually starting in their 70s. The increased dementia risk is independent of sociodemographic, behavioral, cardiometabolic and mental health factors. In other words, chronic sleep deprivation in mid-life, including sleep apnea, is associated with increased risk for development of late-onset dementia.

Studies conducted by researchers of Mayo Clinic and presented in May 2019 to the American Academy of Neurology's 71st Annual Meeting revealed that people who stop breathing during sleep could have high accumulation of the toxic tau protein, one of the two biological hallmarks of Alzheimer's disease. There is more and more scientific evidence to support an association between an increased risk of dementia and sleep disruption, particularly, Obstructive Sleep Apnea (OSA).

According to the recent Study of Aging, Mayo Clinic researchers identified 268 participants aged 65 and older who did not have dementia. Fifteen percent, or 43 of the 268 study participants had bed-partners who witnessed sleep apnea. The participants with witnessed apnea has higher levels of tau, about 5.5%, in the entorhinal cortex than those who have not been observed to have sleep apnea.

PET brain scans revealed buildup of the toxic tau protein in the entorhinal cortex, which is deep behind the nose and susceptible to tau accumulation. The entorhinal cortex stores and retrieves information related to visual perception and when experiences occur. The dysfunctional tau proteins form tangles in such areas of the brain of people with Alzheimer's disease, leading to cognitive decline.

Sleep apnea is a serious sleep disorder; it has three main types:

- Obstructive Sleep Apnea (OSA) --- this is the more common form in which the muscles in the back of the throat relax, unable to support the soft palate, uvula, the tonsils and the tongue. When these muscles relax, the airway closes with inhaling, thus, compromising the air flow and decreasing oxygen levels in the blood, especially to the brain
- Central Sleep Apnea --- this occurs when the brain does not or cannot send proper signals to the muscles that control breathing
- Complex Sleep Apnea Syndrome --- it happens to people affected with both the Obstructive Sleep Apnea and the Central Sleep Apnea

Let us look at the common symptoms of sleep apnea in general:

1. Loud snoring. Spouse, or bed partner even notices dramatic episodes of gasping and struggling to breathe sometimes
2. Morning headaches
3. Lack of energy or feeling exhausted all the time
4. Waking up with dry mouth or sore throat
5. Sleepiness or falling asleep constantly, such as dozing off in a movie theater, or passing out while watching TV on the couch. This can cause deadly consequences because you can fall asleep while driving or performing important tasks
6. Poor memory. You will notice that you will have difficulty remembering simple things like names of friends, what you did just a few minutes ago, and sometimes even what you just ate. All of these seemingly benign memory impairments

happen because your body did not have adequate sleep and did not get into the alpha waves of the sleep cycle which kept you focused and alert during the day
7. Decreased libido (loss of interest in sex)
8. Irritability and mood changes. You may get riled up, frustrated or disgusted over small things that never used to bother you
9. Poor concentration and poor focus. This is because your brain never has chance to recover due to exhaustion from not getting enough deep restful sleep

If you or your loved one is aware of any of the above-mentioned symptoms, seek professional consultation and help as soon as possible to avoid continuing harmful effects on your general and brain health.

Chronic subdural hematoma:

In lay person's term, a subdural hematoma is a collection of blood that accumulates inside the skull but outside the brain. The bleeding occurs within the layers of tissue that surround the brain. Since the skull is not flexible; it does not expand, and any buildup of blood inside it can quickly put pressure on the brain tissues. When the amount of blood underneath the dura, which is the brain's outer wrapper, accumulates large enough, the pressure inside the head can lead to brain damages, unconsciousness, and even death.

Chronic subdural hematoma is a leading cause of reversible dementia, and this condition can result from mild to moderate head trauma unknowingly. It is expected to affect at least 60,000 new individuals in the U.S. by 2030. The elderly people are especially vulnerable because it can occur spontaneously, or they are on medications for anti-coagulation, and not necessarily from a fall or tripping bumping the head or whiplash during a motor vehicle accident. Oftentimes, the sudden impact shaking the skull or sudden shifting of the brain within the skull can tear the tiny blood vessels that bridge between the skull and the brain. Bear in mind that the incidents do not have to be direct blows to the head; in fact, about

50% of the patients with chronic subdural hematoma who report having fallen did so without hitting their heads.

Subdural hematomas are classified based on how fast the blood accumulates:

- Acute subdural hematomas – usually appearing within 72 hours of a traumatic event.
- Subacute subdural hematomas – these are found within 3 to 7 days of an injury.
- Chronic subdural hematomas – these may take weeks or months to appear. They are more commonly seen in the elderly population where brain shrinkage stretches the blood vessels between the skull and brain.

Chronic subdural hematomas are sometimes difficult to diagnose because their symptoms can resemble many other conditions. Ironically, up to 40% of chronic SDH's among the elderly were misdiagnosed as dementia at the time of hospital admission. The following list of symptoms may occur alone or in combination:

- Persistent headache – the most common complaint in SDH patients
- Confusion
- Weakness on one side of the body.
- Drowsiness and/or lethargy
- Visual problems such as diplopia (double vision)
- Problems with balancing or walking
- Slurred speech
- Behavioral and personality changes
- Apathy
- Memory loss or difficulty recalling
- Seizures
- Loss of consciousness

Preventing falls and head injuries, even minor ones, is the most effective way to prevent SDH and the damage it can cause.

Using safety equipment such as seat belts, bicycle helmets and walking canes considerably helps to reduce the risk. Older people in particular must be careful to avoid falls, and make sure your vision is not compromised. Time is of the essence. Early detection and intervention are critical and essential for limiting and reducing lasting damages. Cognitive impairment is the most common symptom in the elderly with chronic subdural hematomas, and usually noticeable in the early phase of the disorder, as opposed to dementia associated with neurodegenerative diseases. So, early neuro-imaging evaluation is important to allow for timely treatment in order to avoid a poor outcome.

After development of chronic subdural hematoma, the brain atrophy rate in the affected elderly is increased to more than twice that of dementia patients without chronic SDH, with a 30% one year mortality rate-an astounding figure!

Brain tumor-associated dementia:

The United States incidence rate for primary brain and nervous system tumors in adults, aged 20 years or older, is estimated to be 23.8 per 100,000 persons. The Central Brain Tumor Registry of the U.S. includes both benign and malignant lesions in its data collected. According to the statistics, about one third of the tumors are malignant and the remainder, or the majority of them are benign. The incidence rate for children is much lower

Brain tumors can also be caused when cancers in other parts of the body spread to the brain. According to the U.S. Central Brain Tumor Registry, approximately 87,000 new cases of primary malignant and non-malignant brain and other CNS tumors will be diagnosed in the United States in 2019. One critical part of the risk to treat brain tumors is to determine how difficult it is to reach the tumor and its location, thus there is no guarantee that a brain tumor is operable.

Brain tumor-associated dementias have features common to other dementias, but also have some unusual characteristics that made a diagnosis of neuro-degenerative disease less likely. The common features include intellectual decline involving difficulties in finding words, the occurrence of paraphasia, poor concentration and focusing, disorientation in familiar surroundings, problems performing routine complex tasks, and social disconnection and withdrawal. Unlike the more common degenerative dementias, however, there is generally no marked memory involvement.

Depending on the locations of brain tumors, there is a wide range of symptoms and warning signs:

- Drowsiness
- Headaches
- Communication difficulty with dysphasia the most common
- Nausea and/or vomiting
- Loss of balance
- Difficulties in routine activities like reading and talking
- Changes in senses like taste and smell (anosmia)
- Papilledema – edema or swelling in the optic disc
- Muscle weakness or paralysis in a certain part of the body
- Visual problems – blurred vision, complete or partial loss of vision
- Bladder control problems
- Mood fluctuations with changes in personality and behavior
- Altered cognition – patients or their family and friends notice that "something is off"
- Memory impairment (difficulties in retaining, recalling and maintaining information)
- Seizures – Up to 60% of patients with brain tumors will experience this at some point, with or without loss of consciousness
- Secretion from the breasts – release of milk is stimulated by a hormone called prolactin. It is synthesized and released in the brain and may be produced by a tumor called prolactinoma growing in the pituitary gland.

There is no doubt that cognitive dysfunction with its impairment permeates the lives of patients suffering from brain tumor from diagnosis to death. It dramatically affects the outcome and quality of their life; it is a heart-breaking dilemma for anyone between survival and dying with dignity. It is of paramount importance for anyone experiencing sudden changes of cognitive functions to go through a complete evaluation!

Environment and Dementia:

Ingestion of toxic substances, which can be described as unintentional poisoning, and environmental exposure to air pollutants can lead to brain damage and eventually, the onset of dementia, according to many recent studies. Chronic Ingestion pf heavy metals or acute exposure to carbon monoxide can lead to toxic encephalopathy, a prelude to dementia. The brain damage is sometimes treatable and reparable, but in cases in which the damage persists, the risk for the development of degenerative dementia greatly increases without a cure.

Heavy metals such as mercury, arsenic, toluene and lithium, even in small doses, can have long-term detrimental effects on the brain, leading to both encephalopathy and dementia. Alcohol, widely available and socially acceptable unfortunately, in excessive or abusive quantities can cause severe, sometimes irreversible damage to the brain. Cyad, with consumable seeds from plants in the Western Pacific, when ingested it can cause neurodegenerative disorders. Any toxic materials, even in minute amounts , especially over a long period of time, can cause gradual mental deterioration.

The symptoms of dementia from toxic substances are very similar to most forms of neurodegenerative dementia, and may include:

- Cognitive impairment
- Memory loss
- Some changes in personality and behavior
- Unexplained fatigue
- Light-headedness or dizziness
- Headache
- Nausea, maybe vomiting in acute cases

- Difficulty in concentration
- Depression

Air pollution has been known for quite some time to cause heart disease and stroke, lung diseases such as asthma, emphysema, lung cancer, chronic obstructive pulmonary disease (COPD), and even early death. One study in China estimated that for the elderly age 75 and over, there are 1166 early deaths for every 100,000 people.

Several other studies from several countries in different continents have linked air pollution to cognitive impairment. Researchers from the study in China found that long-term or chronic exposure to air pollution is associated with poor performance on both verbal and mathematic tests. Moreover, the poor performance on the verbal tests was more pronounced for the older individuals.

Researchers in London, England, found that adults living with the highest annual concentration of air pollution had the highest risk of dementia – 1.4 times the risk of those living with the lowest annual concentration. Researchers from the United States, including the University of Southern California and Harvard Medical School, studied data from 998 women aged 73 to 87 who had both the cognitive tests MRI brain scans, and published their findings in 2020. They revealed two remarkable differences: Cognitively, those exposed to more air pollution showed greater decline in learning a list of words. Anatomically, they showed more cerebral atrophy (shrinkage) in those areas of the brain typically shrink due to Alzheimer's disease, when compared to study participants who were exposed to less air pollution.

Researchers in the above-mentioned studies controlled for every possible confounding factors including sociodemographic factors (age, geographic regions, race/ethnicity, income and education), employment status, clinical history, MRI findings.

The researchers from three different continents came to similar conclusions and believed that " Higher levels of air pollution are associated with a greater risk of cognitive decline, dementia in general and Alzheimer's disease in particular ". This is not to say that air pollution is the direct cause of cognitive decline, but I believe the correlation is real and should not be ignored. According to the U.S. National Institute of Health, both air pollution and dementia are current and growing global issues.

According to a large study of nurses in their 70s, the researchers suggested that smog and other air pollutants can contribute to memory loss and dementia. Furthermore, research conducted over the two decades has provided convincing evidence the role of the natural surroundings – air pollution – may be a significant contributor to dementia. Indeed, exposure to high levels of air pollutants can wreak havoc on your brain!

Some of the most troubling and disturbing studies connecting air pollution to Alzheimer's disease have been conducted in Mexico City, Mexico. One of the findings revealed that adults and children in Mexico City had increased brain expression of beta-amyloid 42, a protein fragment that may contribute to the breakdown of neural communication early in the disease process. The young adults and children in areas of high levels of air pollutants had both amyloid plaque and tau pathology, where as the children and young adults in the control groups had neither of the abnormal proteins. Moreover, the participants in the Mexico study also showed many other abnormalities that are common features in other neurodegenerative diseases.

Another study in Taiwan with more than 92,000 subjects found a dose-dependent relationship between how much air pollution levels increased in a particular region and the risk of residents within that region developing dementia, specifically, Alzheimer's disease, with each 10,91 parts per billion increase in ozone, a common measure of air pollution that results from automobile emissions and industrial wastes. There are also other types of air pollutants in the atmosphere such as gases, particulates, and biological molecules.

All these studies suggest the negative and harmful effects on our general health, mental health in particular, living in areas with high levels of air pollution, and its potential real life consequences of cognitive decline and dementia. Directly or indirectly, we are all responsible for air pollution in our cities, our nation, and our planet. WE ALL SHOULD DO OUR PARTS TO REDUCE OUR CARBON FOOTPRINT.

Certain lifestyle changes will also help lower air pollution levels in our communities, such as carpooling and limiting the use of gas-powered lawn care equipment during the hottest hours of the day, just to name a few. Reducing, and avoiding air pollution, if you can, may be a long-term, worthwhile investment that your brain will thank you for. From the perspectives of the development of dementia, there are other environmental factors including , but not limited to, physical activities (walking and exercise), nutrition (balanced and plant-based diet), mental stimulations (learning and using new information), adequate sleep, healthy habits, and positive social relationships.

According to researchers at Boston University School of Public Health, they studied more than 13,500 women with an average age of 61 and found that clean air and greenery with plants and flowers decreased depression and the risk of developing dementia. This should not be a surprise because exposure to parks, forest preserve, community gardens and other green space is relaxing and de-stressing along with socializing with friends outside, mitigating the risk of dementia. Policy makers and city-planners should consider this as a potential population-level approach to improve cognitive health.

Wernicke-Korsakoff Syndrome:

This is a common complication of thiamine (vitamin B1) deficiency, primarily seen with alcoholics. It is actually a combination of two medical conditions in the brain caused by thiamine deficiency: Wernicke's encephalopathy and Korsakoff psychosis. Some scientists suggest that the syndrome represents a continuum, with Wernicke's encephalopathy as the acute phase of the disorder while Korsakoff psychosis progressing to a long-lasting stage with permanent brain damage.

Wernicke's encephalopathy, a degenerative brain disorder, usually results from alcohol abuse, other causes may include dietary deficiency, prolonged vomiting, eating disorders, or side-effects of chemotherapy. This acute, neurological condition is characterized by a clinical triad of ophthalmoparesis with nystagmus, ataxia, and confusion. Most of the symptoms can be reversed if detected early and treated promptly. Delayed treatment can lead to severe morbidity and mortality; the prophylactic thiamine administration is relatively safe, and should be initiated and instituted even before the diagnosis is confirmed.

In the Korsakoff's amnesic syndrome or psychosis, neurons and the brain's supporting cells are damaged and symptoms include amnesia, tremor, disorientation, vision problems, and coma. The memory impairment leads to problems in acquiring new information, in retrieving previous memories, and establishing new memories.

In thiamine deficiency, people at risk besides alcoholics, include the malnutrition-prone homeless people, older and vagrant individuals, and people living alone or in isolation, and patients with psychiatric conditions. It can also occur in women during the first trimester of pregnancy with hyperemesis gravidarum. In addition to timely thiamine replacement, proper nutritional support and hydration must be provided. There are more than 200,000 cases per year in the U.S. Sadly, the prognosis of Wernicke-Korsakoff Syndrome is poor, and the mortality rate of Wernicke Encephalopathy can be as high as 20%, and about 80% of the affected patients survive and progress to Korsakoff psychosis.

Certain infections and their incident dementia:

Dementia-like symptoms can result from febrile illness or other side effects of the body's attempt to fight off an infection in an acute setting. The infected persons may develop thinking difficulties from a urinary tract infection, meningitis, encephalitis, Lyme disease, HIV and AIDS, and syphilis. It is possible to overlook in the case of syphilis because cognitive changes usually appear in later stages of the disease.

Some of the infections are curable, such as urinary tract infections; though cognitive impairment or dementia caused by an infection is not very common, but it is an important step in the evaluation of anyone suspected of having dementia symptoms or any changes in cognitive functioning.

The recent and on-going pandemic of COVID-19 has upended many lives and changed many policies globally. Many studies seem to have suggested that the Covid infections may increase a person's risk for the development of dementia, and some experts already predict a spike in dementia cases with the long Covid-19 pandemic. As of the start of year 2022, more than 35 million Americans have tested positive for COVID-19, and global Coronavirus cases have already topped 200 million, according to the World Health Organization (WHO).

A recent report from the Alzheimer's Association states that deaths from Alzheimer's disease were about 16% higher in 2020 than in previous years, and most of the increased deaths can be attributed to COVID-19. Over the long term, researchers have suggested that the number of people with dementia could rise significantly due to the neurological impact of COVID-19. The unsettled and serious effects of the so-called ' long Covid ' cannot be ignored or taken lightly, and the CNS symptoms include the loss of taste and smell, brain fog, and difficulties with concentration, memory and thinking.

One study, in fact, found that as many as 1 in 3 COVID-19 survivors experience a mental health or neurological disorder within six months of a coronavirus infection. Another study discovered that nearly half of patients hospitalized with COVID-19 had suffered negative changes in brain function or structure. It is incontrovertible that the disease burden and costs associated with dementia, including medical care and expenses, will certainly rise stupendously. Based on one estimate by the World Health Organization, it will reach $2.8 trillion annually by 2030!

Post-operative Delirium and Dementia

Post-surgical delirium is a common, if not the most common complication in older adults after an operation, and ironically, it is often undiagnosed. By definition, delirium is a serious disruption in one's mental functions that results in unclear or confused thinking with some cognitive impairments. Other symptoms include reduced awareness of the surroundings or absence of response to the environment, restlessness and anxiety, incoherence, and hallucination (seeing things that do not exist). Sometimes, the affected person can experience difficulty speaking or recalling words, reading or writing. Other noticeable symptoms include trouble understanding speech, personality and/or mood changes, and memory impairment, especially for recent events.

Three types of delirium have been identified:

- Hyperactive delirium with agitation, restlessness, irritability, combativeness, and sometimes hallucination
- Hypoactive delirium with lethargy, sluggishness, drowsiness and reduced motor activities
- Mixed delirium with both hyper- and hypo-active states. The affected person may switch back and forth from hyperactive to hypoactive states

There are several contributing and causative factors to post-surgical delirium:

- Infection

- Drugs
- Sensory deprivations (blindness and deafness)
- Alcohol intoxication or withdrawal
- Electrolyte imbalance
- Immobilization (unable to move around)

Post-surgical delirium can last only a few hours, a few days, or as long as several weeks or months. The extent of recovery depends on the health and mental status of the patients before the onset of delirium. People with history of dementia, for example, may experience an overall significant decline in memory and thinking skills. People in better health status are more likely to fully recover.

According to the most recent statistics from the American Hospital Association, about 4 to 5 adults in the U.S. hospitals become delirious every minute after surgeries under general anesthesia. These high figures are astounding, adding up to about 2.5 million cases of post-surgical delirium annually. Many medical professionals regard post-surgical delirium as a ' normal ' but temporary state with little or without any long-term impact because the symptoms are generally short-lived. This opinion is debatable and superficial because some older patients could not even remember their birthdays or what country they were in beyond the three-four days after surgeries. Researchers noticed that many, with follow-up studies, showed continued decline of their cognitive abilities with a diagnosis of Alzheimer's disease one year after the ' incident' of post-surgical delirium.

We must honestly admit that post-surgical delirium is probably more prevalent than people realize, and should not minimize its profound impact on brain health. Unfortunately, the causes for the observed symptoms in post-surgical delirium are not clear at this time due to multi-causality and multi-dimensionality of this medical phenomena. General anesthesia during surgery may play a role according to some researchers. Patients became unconscious under general anesthesia, but in post-anesthetic unconscious state, the neurons of different senses do not stop firing and their activities can be demonstrated in brain-wave studies. In reality and actuality, patients' neuronal connectivities are subdued or suppressed during sedation by general anesthesia. During post-operative recovery, most patients were able to resume normal brain activities, but in some post-op patients, I believe that the connectivities in their brains are compromised.

In addition to the possible adverse effects of general anesthesia, anxiety in general as a reaction to the surgical procedure, along with post-operative medications, such as opioid analgesics and sedatives, may be involved. Furthermore, any unsuspected, pre-existing neurodegenerative disorders can be a major risk factor for the development of post-surgical delirium. Nevertheless, the current statistics for the high number of cases are just mind-boggling and hard to accept passively. Healthcare providers must all strive to reduce and avoid if possible, the incidents of post-surgical delirium, and not to consider and accept them as temporary complications after surgeries, because these cases can have far-reaching, devastating effects on the suffering patients and their families, and the society as a whole.

Immediate attention should be focused on patients' post-operative nutritional support, the avoidance of mind-altering medications if possible, appropriate and continued brain stimulations for the senses such as eye-glasses and hearing aids, and their surroundings which promote safe, restful sleep (environmental support).

Before contemplating any major surgery requiring general anesthesia, it is important that patient and family should convene including attending physician and designated surgeon to discuss the risks and types of anesthesia for the surgical procedure, especially an elective operation. The attending anesthesiologist or anesthetist ideally should be present at the meeting to educate and answer any questions. More and more medical institutions, including medical schools and hospitals have accepted and used acupunctural anesthesia as an option, if appropriate, for certain surgical procedures. Both patients and family and loved ones should be proactive when considering major surgery under general anesthesia to become educated medical consumers. After all, it is your life, and your brain at risk, and life without a normal, functioning brain is no life at all!

Dr. Richard Ng, B.S., D.O.

For adults, older ones in particular, who are going to have surgeries requiring general anesthesia, a pre-surgical screening along with a mini-mental status examination should ne performed by qualified medical professionals or psychologists to have a baseline study prior to the surgery. Prior to the operation, you should start or continue your healthy lifestyle with regular exercise, proper nutrition and diet, and adequate sleep to prepare yourself for the surgery and to minimize the risk of post-surgical delirium.

Any surgical procedure, especially under general anesthesia, carries some risk, and nobody can guarantee it risk-free; everyone of us should be aware of the possibility of post-surgical delirium and its potential impact on increasing the risk for the development of Alzheimer's disease and/or dementia. Therefore, as an established preventive protocol, a careful and in-depth ore-surgical assessment is crucial with collaboration of the medical team consisting of attending physician, designated surgeon, anesthesiologist or supervised anesthetist, and qualified psychologist, taking any contributing risk factors into consideration.

Signs and Symptoms of Dementia in General

The National Institute on Aging defines dementia as " the loss of cognitive functioning --- thinking, remembering and reasoning --- with disruptive behaviors that interfere with a person's daily life and activities ". Alzheimer's disease or dementia is not an actual consequence of aging or a normal part of aging, even though it primarily affects the older population. According to the Centers for Diseases Control and Prevention (CDC), "dementia is not a specific disease, but a rather general term for the impaired ability to remember, think, or make decisions that interfere with doing everyday activities."

As already mentioned in this book, there are several types of dementia including Alzheimer's disease, vascular dementia, Lewis Body Dementia, and Frontotemporal Dementia to name a few. Alzheimer's disease is the most common type, accounting for about 70% of dementia cases. Globally, more than 50 million people have dementia based on the current statistics, and an estimated 10 million new cases are reported each year. Projections of the World Health Organization (WHO) show that the number of affected individuals will reach 82 million in year 2030 and 152 million by year 2050. The social disease burdens of dementia are horrendous and stupendous; the long-term effects of dementia can be so saddening, heart-breaking and difficult for both those affected and their caregivers, family and friends.

Early diagnosis of dementia is especially important, with myriad of benefits; it can help with planning both at home and at work, with preventive care and other preemptive and supportive measures such as simple reminders. It also enables dementia patients to access clinical trials and available, current therapies that may improve cognitive functioning and overall quality of life.

Unfortunately, an early and timely diagnosis is not the norm or reality for many people living with dementia. Research, in fact, has shown that the average time from when symptoms appear to diagnosis is about three years --- and waiting period could be even longer for those in low-income, disadvantaged and minority communities. Some people, those with lower education levels in particular, may not see a doctor until it's too late for them to plan ahead; they don't recognize the signs and symptoms or they think the signs and symptoms are just a normal part of aging. In fact, fewer than one in five Americans are familiar with early signs or warnings of dementia, or a condition known as cognitive impairment. Up to 70% of primary care providers (PCPs) struggle to distinguish its early symptoms from the so-called normal aging, according to a report released by the Alzheimer's Association.

Another benefit of an earlier diagnosis is patient-centered, allowing patients to plan ahead and have more input over their future, if they have an accurate diagnosis early on. Undoubtedly, people with dementia need a multidisciplinary, time-intensive model with a focus on early diagnosis and treatment. With insufficient funding and Medicare reimbursement, inadequate education of physicians and laypeople, a shortage of geriatricians, and lack of communication among caregivers, patients, and their healthcare providers are all contributing to a delay in diagnosis and subsequent appropriate care that will have a significant, lasting impact on the health and finance of society. It is in our best interest to overcome the barriers to an early diagnosis in dementia!

With your high index of suspicion, early diagnosis of dementia is worth the risk of offending a loved one. Let us look at the early signs and symptoms of dementia with the start of a day in the morning:

- While it may seem like a simple task for us to get dressed in the morning independently, this act actually involves planning and many steps. The damage dementia inflicts on the brain of the affected person can cause confusion in these routines. They may wear the same clothes day after day, probably, the person with dementia finds comfort and security in the familiar outfit. People with impaired executive functioning of the brain (decision-making) may dress for the wrong season due to limited judgment and possible poor self-regulation of body temperature. The impaired person may put on their pants first and forget to wear the underwear. The affected person may put on their clothes backwards. Or, he or she forgets the steps needed to put on a shirt or a jacket, such as putting an arm through the piece of clothing or uneven buttoning.

- Forgetting recently learned information repeatedly, not remembering important dates and events, asking the same question several times or repeating the same stories again and again because they simply cannot remember what said or did just minutes before. Many have difficulty to recall or recognize familiar people or familiar objects, although vision has not been compromised; this is certainly far beyond simple forgetfulness and the so-called ' senior moments'. Of course, some of these things may be due to ' mild cognitive impairment ', but not always. Memory loss can also be a sign of depression, vitamin B12 deficiency, brain disease, thyroid disorder, or a side-effect of certain medications.
- Every person with dementia will experience this unfortunate condition differently. A 2018 study published in the journal Materia Sociomedica says that "difficulties related to communication are among the earliest symptoms of dementia." Language difficulties are a major problem for most of the patients with dementia, essentially throughout the course of the illness from early to late stages. The impaired individuals with dementia may use words that have no meaning, or they are mixed up in the wrong order, a form of aphasia. This can occur occasionally or regularly depending on the severity of the condition.
- Sometimes, the affected person may not be able to find the right words, not finding any word at all, or reverting back to one's first language that was learned as a child. Difficulty

in language expression --- whether oral or written, or understanding a message. The loss of communication is complex, e.g. the person may understand what you say, but unable to express themselves through spoken language. Or they can express themselves, but do not understand what is being said. Or they have difficulties in writing the words. Indeed, the difficulty with language communication experienced by individuals with dementia is broad, including comprehension, reading, spelling and writing. The problems can be very frustrating for the impaired person, the listener should keep the tone as light, positive, and good-humored as possible. This can help relieve tension and bring you closer together, if you are a caregiver.

- Diagnosing dementia is definitely not an easy task, and currently, no single diagnostic test exists for dementia. There are some telltale signs, but many subtle signs and symptoms are easy to ignore. A team of experts at Newcastle University in the United Kingdom report that simply by analyzing a person's gait can help doctors diagnose dementia sooner with more accuracy. Researchers have found that dying and dysfunctional brain cells associated with dementia affect many activities of daily living---not just memory and cognitive skills, but also walking. Scientific evidence has shown that walking patterns change before memory and recognition problems become apparent. So, a noticeable change in a person's pace or gait while he or she walks could be an early sign of dementia. Watch the way your loved one walks, and if he or she starts to show deterioration in their gait and pattern and have no other explanation for it, you need to seek medical advice proactively and pay attention to any memory issues. Research has already proven the connection between gait and dementia.

- The affected person's inability to use common and familiar hand tools and trouble to operate familiar appliances at home can be a ' red flag '

- Challenges in routine management of household finances, like paying bills with checks, or planning such as following recipes used for years.
- Withdrawal from work or social activities, probably due to apathetic behavior. For example, stop or not wanting to go to church with the family and not interested in watching favorite sports on TV because the affected person cannot keep up with what is going on.
- Misplacing things and losing the ability to retrace the steps to find them, such as placing car keys in the washer or dryer, or putting the wallet in the refrigerator.
- The person with dementia can get confused with time or place, such as losing track of dates, or not recognizing the location. Thus, they tend to be wandering slowly and purposelessly.
- Frequent falls and trips are not uncommon partially due to the affected person's impaired visuo-spatial functions. They have problem understanding visual images and spatial relations, i.e. they find it difficult to perceive an object's position in relation to others or themselves. In other words, they have difficulty with balance and judging distance. Some may have poor posture control and difficulty planning and executing the movements. Thus, you will often see your loved one with dementia tripping over things at home, or spilling or dropping things.
- Not understanding sarcasm – there may be an impaired function of the dorsolateral portion of the frontal lobes, where assessment of emotional meanings take place. The affected person just cannot understand the implicit content of sarcasm. This is analogous to appreciation of and laughing at a funny joke.
- Loss of empathy – the affected person loses interest in what happens around them, and this often leads to social isolation worsening the condition, and withdrawal from work.
- The affected person, even known to be good-natured and mild-tempered, can show changes in mood and personality, getting easily upset and angry in common situations.

- People suffering from dementia do not seem to take joy in life's simple pleasures such as their favorite meals, or hilarious, funny sitcom on TV. This withdrawal from enjoyed activities can be one of the early signs of dementia. This lack of or impaired ability to experience pleasure, called anhedonia, is discovered by a recent study conducted at the University of Sidney in Australia of patients diagnosed of Fronto-Temporal Dementia (FTD).
- Napping too much during the day in older adults could be a worrying warning sign of dementia. A team of researchers in the U.S. have found that excessive napping in the day increased the risk of Alzheimer's and dementia, while both conditions also caused old people to take more naps during the daytime. It is the amount of the nap and its pattern that deserve the attention. A short nap of 10 to 15 minutes in a hectic day can be refreshing and rejuvenating.

Signs and symptoms of dementia are multiple and variable, to say the least. The affected person may notice some of the signs and symptoms themselves, but their family members or caregivers may notice others. WHO (world health organization) divides dementia into roughly three stages:

- Early stage – the affected person become more forgetful, feel lost in familiar places, and lose track of time.
- Middle stage – symptoms become more noticeable with forgetting names and recent events. Affected person may feel lost even at home and has difficulty communicating; they show more noticeable behavioral changes.
- Late stage – the affected person needs full-time assistance. They are unaware of where they are. They are unaware of time. They have difficulty recognizing people including loved ones. Walking becomes more and more difficult that they become more and more bedridden. Obvious behavioral changes which may include aggression.

Factors that increase the risk of dementia

According to the Lancet Commission's 2020 report on dementia prevention, intervention, and care, they have 12 factors on their list that can decrease the risk of certain type of dementia, or delay its onset, or simply prevent it. Together, the Lancet Commission reports that the twelve risk factors account for about 40% of dementias worldwide. This is significant and encouraging; however, we can add a few other modifiable risk factors which include chronic sleep deprivation, poor vision and non-plant-based diet.

Here is the list from the Lancet Commission's 2020 report on dementia:

1. Less education
2. Hypertension
3. Hearing impairment
4. Smoking
5. Obesity
6. Depression
7. Physical inactivity
8. Diabetes
9. Low levels or lack of social contact
10. Alcohol consumption
11. Traumatic Brain Injury (TBI)
12. Air pollution (chronic exposure)

The items in the list are modifiable factors and their positive changes are neuro-protective, reducing the risk of developing dementia, with a plethora of scientific evidence. Dementia is not a death sentence, and it is possible to delay its onset and mitigate its scourge to improve the quality of life of both the affected individuals and caregivers, and hopefully forestalling it with all of our worthwhile efforts.

Less Education
– Lower education level, in general, is associated with less cognitive reserve. According to many studies, some of the remarkable reductions in the risk of developing Alzheimer's disease have been linked to higher levels of education --- with each year of schooling beyond elementary levels considerably increasing the overall neuroprotective benefits. Furthermore, intellectual activities and late-life learning are well known and proven by researchers to offer protection from Alzheimer's disease and dementia. In 2017, a group of European researchers studied the data of more than 55,000 people and found that their risk of dementia dropped with each completed year of formal education. Advances in education with mentally enriched and challenging environments, coupled with improvements in health care and living conditions could explain their lower rates of Alzheimer's disease and dementia.

According to neuroscientific research, the mental stimulation in an enriched, challenging environment promotes the development of new neurons and connections to expand the brain reserve. It is encouraging to know that education is a neuroprotective factor, this is not to say that if you do not have higher education beyond elementary levels, you are doomed to get and suffer from Alzheimer's disease and dementia. In fact, there are many things one can do and pursue in the learning processes to stimulate brain activities, leading to more active and more abundant dendritic branches and axonal terminals --- arborization. Here are some suggestions:

- Learning a new language
- Learning to play a new musical instrument
- Learning a new skill or craft
- Reading a book and looking up the dictionary for the new vocabularies

- Reading story books to your grand-children
- Playing non-violent video games and grabbing that joystick. Studies have found that this stimulates the parts of the brain that control movements, memory, planning and fine motor skills
- Doing numbers and word puzzles are a great way to maintain your cognitive edge. They are also a fun way to spend time with people you like and to bond with family and friends
- Playing chess, cards, or mahjong (Mahjong is a Chinese game playing with marked, small rectangular tiles on a special table. The four players shuffle and move the tiles randomly with a specific position for each player, ease, south, west or north. This game involves a lot of mental stimulation and physical activities of the arms and shoulders.
- Watching TV news, or history/discovery channels, but to cultivate a habit of getting up to move around every 30 minutes to avoid prolonged sitting
- Signing up for a class you like and will enjoy at a community college, non-credit or for credit, and finding yourself in an intellectually stimulating surroundings with social interactions
- Visiting a museum in your city with friends and family to learn something interesting and new, while getting some exercise at a leisurely pace.

Even though limited schooling may be a negative factor in terms of neuroprotection, it is your choice and within your power to overcome the pre-existing disadvantages and to invest in your future for optimal brain health. The adult brains do make new neurons, when given the right, stimulating environments --- adult neurogenesis. Neuroplasticity and the ability of neuronal arborization of the brain make it possible to achieve neuroprotection against mental decline, to slow down or halt the progression of Alzheimer's disease and certain types of dementia. It is indisputable that late life learning and intellectual activities offer protection from and reduce the risk of Alzheimer's disease and dementia. It seems almost as if Nature says "we know you are not physically strong enough to contribute to society as a work-horse at this juncture of life, but we still value your wisdom and intellect. If you are not using your brain, then perhaps it is time to bow out". Just remember a proverbial saying: " Use it or lose it ".

Hypertension
--- High blood pressure is a common condition that will catch up with most people who live into older age. In contrast to the relatively high prevalence of high blood pressure in the U.S., many non-westernized and developing countries and remote populations have a low prevalence of hypertension and do not experience an increase in blood pressure with age in general. Approximately, 30% of the American adults have the diagnosis of hypertension; furthermore, about another 30% of the adult U.S. population have pre-hypertension. Hypertension is sometimes called " a silent killer " because it may have no obvious symptoms for years. In most cases, the underlying causes of high blood pressure are unknown, essential or idiopathic, but many people with the diagnosis have identifiable correctable conditions. Hypertension is indeed a major global health concern, and a primary risk factor for cardiovascular disease, including stroke, heart attack and aneurysm.

If high blood pressure is ignored and left untreated, overtime, it can quietly cause far-reaching damage to the heart, lungs, blood vessels, kidneys and the brain. It is indisputable that hypertension has serious harmful impact on the microvascular and vascular systems of the body, especially the brain. If your blood pressure remains elevated despite diet, lifestyle and behavioral changes, it is important for you to consult your doctor for professional advice. Data pooled from six large observational studies have suggested that anti-hypertensive medications may lower the risk of Alzheimer's disease and other types of dementia. The review was published in Lancet Neurology in 2019, and the studies involved more than 31,000 participants older than 55 with follow-ups ranging from seven to twenty-two years. Among the 15,537 participants with the diagnosis of hypertension, those using and compliant with the prescribed blood pressure medications had a 12% reduced risk of dementia and 16% reduced risk of developing Alzheimer's disease. The remaining 15,553 participants without history of hypertension had the same risk for dementia as those who controlled their blood pressure with medications.

Hypertension is a major risk factor for premature death, cardiovascular disease and stroke, and stroke is a co-morbidity in up to 30% of Alzheimer's patients, if not higher. For people with diagnosed hypertension, it is very important to take their blood pressure medications faithfully and follow-up with your doctors to minimize the risk of dementia.

The association between hypertension and brain health including dementia in later life has been well-established; however, according to recent findings published in Hypertension, an American Heart Association journal, significant brain changes can be found even among younger individuals with high blood pressure. Researchers looked at health information from about 500,000 volunteer participants in the United Kingdom, including magnetic resonance imaging (MRI) measurements of brain volume. They discovered that both the total brain volume and brain volume in specific regions were smaller in people aged 35 to 50 diagnosed with hypertension than in study participants without high blood pressure. In addition, the researchers found that the risk of dementia was much higher, up to 60%, in people diagnosed with high blood pressure between the ages of 35 and 45 compared with those with normal blood pressure.

There is no quick fix here, and lifestyle adjustments and changes are the standard first-line treatment. There are a few things you can do to improve your high blood pressure such as:

- Reduce sodium intake, a common component of the common table salt
- Reduce your weight if you are overweight
- Reduce alcohol, be a moderate consumer
- Quit cigarette smoking
- Reduce sugar intake, especially if you are diabetic
- Regular exercise, 150 minutes a week

- Reduce stress
- Following the DASH diet (Dietary Approach to Stop Hypertension), as recommended by the U.S. National Heart, Lungs and Blood Institute

Hearing Impairment or Loss

--- Hearing loss doesn't just mean an older adult needs to turn up the TV. In fact, it has been linked to the development of dementia. The latest aging research not only shows the two are connected, it is also leading researchers to believe that hearing loss may actually be a cause of dementia.

Hearing loss is not always related to an underlying medical condition. It may be caused by:

- Cerumen impaction (ear wax accumulation)
- Noise exposure
- Aging
- Severe pressure change
- Ototoxic medications (drugs that damage function of ears)
- Traumatic injuries
- Foreign object inside the ears

There are different types of hearing loss, including but not limited to sensorineural hearing loss, high-frequency hearing loss, and conductive hearing loss. The causes of hearing loss vary from person to person, knowing what is causing it is key to finding the right solution. According to the National Institute on Aging (NIA), about two-thirds of adults age 70 or older have difficulty hearing, because most of us will lose some of our ability to hear as we age. Unfortunately, hearing loss in the geriatric population is often overlooked, according to recently published research.

In a new study published in July 2021 in Alzheimer's & Dementia journal, researchers at the University of Oxford in the UK studied 82,039 men and women aged 60 and older from the U.K. Biobank, by asking participants to identify numbers that were spoken over a background of white noise. Based on the results, each participant was then categorized as having normal, insufficient, or poor hearing. The researchers continued to follow up with the participants for 11 years, finding that 1,285 subjects were eventually diagnosed dementia, based on health and death records. The final analyses showed that those in the ' insufficient hearing ' group had a 61 percent increased risk of developing dementia compared to those with normal hearing, while those in the ' poor hearing ' group saw a startling 91 percent increased risk. The conclusion is: " Not being able to hear during a conversation could mean a higher risk of dementia."

The Royal National Institute for Deaf People states that hearing loss is clearly associated with an increased risk of dementia. Researchers from Northern Ireland studied 2,114 patients, aged over 50, with a hearing impairment, from the National Alzheimer's Co-ordinating Center. The team found that a third of participants who wore hearing aids had not developed dementia five years after the diagnosis of mild cognitive impairment (MCI). In contrast, this figure was only a fifth for those who did not use hearing aids.

There is no doubt that untreated hearing loss can lead to emotional frustration and social isolation, and many older people with hearing impairment may simply become withdrawn. According to the Center for Disease Control and Prevention (CDC), loved ones themselves are usually the first to notice this phenomenon. Hearing plays a large, important role in how we socialize with other people. Early detection and intervention can help improve hearing health and stop worsening hearing loss. Many scientific studies have already demonstrated that untreated hearing loss can increase the risk of memory loss as well as onset of dementia.

Some studies have found that people with moderate hearing loss or poor hearing tended to decline faster in terms of physical function over the six years of observation. This is understandable because most people with impaired hearing tend to be more socially isolated with more sedentary behavior. This is a double whammy: social isolation and decreased physical activity greatly heighten the risk of dementia, or accelerate its onset, let alone with the increased risk of other health problems. Nowadays, hearing loss can be treated successfully with many modalities and options. Be proactive, the sooner the better!

Cigarette Smoking --- many of the harmful effects from cigarette smoking were discussed in previous section of this book. Both smokers and non-smokers are aware of the increased risk of lung cancer associated with cigarette smoking, but unaware of the multiple serious health consequences of smoking. Studies have shown that the chance of premature death from any cause is much higher with smokers as compared with non-smokers, including dying of a heart attack. Chronic obstructive pulmonary disease (COPD) such as emphysema, asthma and bronchitis are more common among smokers. Tobacco use is still the leading cause of preventable death in the United States. According to the Centers for Disease Control and Prevention (CDC), close to a half million Americans die prematurely each year due to smoking or exposure to second-hand smoke.

In addition to the polluted air you breathe and the hundreds of toxic chemicals in every cigarette, smoking is a strong producer of millions of free radicals, causing elevated levels of oxidative stress. In a cascade of chemical chain reaction, inflammatory cells are activated, provoking and resulting in cellular damages. The extensive oxidative stress and accompanying inflammation present a major risk factor for development of cardiovascular disease, cancer, and neurodegenerative disorders like Alzheimer's disease. The most notorious harmful chemical in cigarette is nicotine, which is highly addictive and a powerful vasoconstrictor. Its property of vasoconstriction can increase blood pressure and decrease blood flow which carries nutrients and oxygen, elevating the risk of stroke directly and the risk for the development of Alzheimer's disease indirectly with micro-hemorrhages of the brain.

There is a strong evidence that smoking can increase your risk of developing dementia. Not everyone who smokes will get dementia, but stopping will reduce your risk down to the level of non-smokers. Smoking remains a leading cause of premature death, and many smokers, especially regular, heavy smokers, are likely to die before they reach the age at which dementia will develop. According to research, the two most common forms of dementia, Alzheimer's and vascular dementia, have been linked to problems with the vascular system. The World Alzheimer's Report 2014 examined the findings from seven systemic reviews and they also carried out their own. A total of 14 studies were included in this large review, and the researchers found that there was statistically significant increases risk of dementia in smokers compared to people who have never smoked.

According to a 2012 study, researchers examined the cognitive data of more than 7,000 men and women over a 12-year period, and found that middle-aged male smokers experienced more rapid cognitive decline than non-smokers. Furthermore, the longer their smoking history, the higher their risk of bigger, age-related brain volume loss. Most people understand how smoking affects the heart and lungs, but unaware of the impact that nicotine has on the brain. Thus, by quitting cigarette smoking, you have everything to gain, including your heart, your lungs and your brain.

Depression --- it is a mood disorder that causes a persistent feeling of sadness and loss of interest. Depression is a risk factor for dementia, according to researchers at the Rush University Alzheimer's Disease Center, and with more symptoms of depression tend to suffer more rapid decline in thinking and memory skills. While many studies found an association between the two, it did not prove a cause-and-effect relationship. Common symptoms of depression include:

- Sadness which is persistent
- Fatigue
- Difficulty concentrating and focusing
- Profound anger
- Irritability
- Easy frustration
- Loss of interest in pleasurable or fun activities
- Sleep issues, either too much or too little
- Lack of energy
- Anxiety, usually inexplicable
- Social isolation

Both depression and dementia are common diseases; depression can occur during any stage of life, while dementia usually occurs during later stages of life. Many studies have shown that depression can lead to dementia, and it can have a profound and significant impact on those already suffering from dementia. Whether depression comes before or after the diagnosis of dementia remains unclear, but there is a clear connection between the two diseases.

Depression in the elderly can often lead to a phenomenon called pseudodementia – an apparent intellectual decline that arises from a lack of energy or effort. People with this condition are usually forgetful, moving slowly, and having low motivation as well as mental slowing. This condition responds well to treatments for depression. As their mood improves, the individual's energy, ability to focus and concentrate, and intellectual functioning oftentimes return to their previous levels.

Mental illness in early life is associated with an increased risk of dementia in later years. Results of a large longitudinal, population-based study show that individuals hospitalized for a mental health disorder had a fourfold increased risk for developing dementia compared to those who were not hospitalized with a mental illness. Supporting younger people's mental health could be a window of opportunity to help reduce the burden, or delay the onset of dementia in older adults. Anyway, if you suspect that someone you love who suffers from dementia may be becoming depressed, it is imperative to consult the physician or a medical professional as soon as possible for appropriate treatment plan, because an untreated depression can become a serious health hazard, and depression is indeed a modifiable risk factor for dementia.

Diabetes --- It is so prevalent worldwide, not just in the U.S.; unfortunately many people don't even know that they are diabetic or pre-diabetic. In general, to be in the healthy range, blood glucose levels should be lower than 100 mg/dl, with measurements from 100-125 mg/dl considered pre-diabetic. Type-2 diabetes is more prevalent in our modern society than ever before, leading to an overall 5% increase in premature deaths since 2000. It is particularly troublesome because type-2 diabetes is now being seen frequently in children, due to their inactivity and obesity.

Today, the average American consumes at least 80 pounds of added sugar annually, or about 22 to 25 teaspoons of added sugar daily! Poor control of blood sugar is the hallmark of diabetes mellitus. Hyperglycemia or excess sugar reacts with proteins to form Advanced Glycation End-products (AGEs), which are actually oxidation products, blocking normal functioning and altering the structures of the protein molecules. Studies have shown that the glycated hemoglobin becomes sticky when there is too much sugar in the blood, resulting in the production of AGEs. When AGEs form in the brain, the sticky damaged neurons can no longer transmit electrical impulses effectively, disrupting memories, thus increasing the risk of Alzheimer's disease. Please be reminded that almost any molecules in the body in the milieu of hyperglycemia can suffer the same fate with AGEs.

According to the Centers for Disease Control and Prevention, the vast majority of people with diabetes have type-2, which becomes more common in older people, as does dementia. Insulin resistance does not develop overnight, it occurs over many years when the body cannot properly utilize the insulin it makes to control blood sugar levels. Most people know that diabetes is unhealthy, affecting many organs of the body including the cardiovascular systems and the kidneys. Blood sugar control is also very important for maintaining good and healthy brain. Normal blood glucose levels are critical for brain health. The brain is about 2% of the body's weight, but it uses 20% to 30% of the circulating blood sugar. Clearly, the brain is a big user of the body's glucose supply. Since the brain does not store excess glucose, that inherently makes it vulnerable to the highs and lows of blood glucose levels. In fact, many researchers believe that the increased risk for the development of dementia among diabetic patients is linked to highs and lows in the body's blood sugar levels.

When there is too little sugar in the blood, the brain does not have the levels of energy it needs to perform tasks; essentially, the brain is being starved during hypoglycemic episodes.

Patients with diabetes are at risk for early-onset dementia and mortality, especially among the middle-age group, according to researchers in Australia. The researchers at Curtin University conducted a retrospective study using Western Australian hospital in-patients, mental health out-patients and death records to compare the age of dementia onset and survival outcomes among dementia patients with and without pre-existing diabetes. According to the findings, dementia onset occurred at an average of 2.2 years and death 2.6 years earlier in patients when compared with patients without diabetes. The public health significance of a 2.2- year age difference may seem modest and insignificant, yet it has been estimated that any intervention to delay the onset of Alzheimer's disease by 2.2 years would reduce the projected tripling or quadrupling of Alzheimer's disease prevalence by year 2050 by 20%. These significant and meaningful findings have major implications for calculating the future Alzheimer's burden due to diabetes, a modifiable risk factor, as well as clinical impacts for the affected patients and their families.

The importance of the linkage between type-2 diabetes and Alzheimer's dementia is perhaps best described by the term " type-3 diabetes ", referring to some patients who develop Alzheimer's disease dementia as a result of diabetes-related damage and degeneration in the brain.

Beta amyloid protein fragments and excess insulin are degraded and cleared by the Insulin Degrading Enzymes (IDE) in a normal equilibrium. However, when hyper-insulinemia becomes chronic, the IDE will prioritize to clear the insulin, allowing the beta amyloid to accumulate. Studies have shown that when blood insulin levels are low, such as a low carbohydrate diet, more beta amyloid proteins are degraded and cleared by the IDE. In other words, a low-carbohydrate diet can be protective against Alzheimer's disease, especially in patients with diabetes.

Physical Inactivity
--- Sedentary lifestyle or physical inactivity is hazardous to your health, including the brain. Getting in a daily dose of exercise can be as simple as going out for a walk. I just cannot emphasize enough about the importance of walking as part of your lifestyle, especially for individuals suffering from Alzheimer's disease in their early stages. The early stage of this neurodegenerative disorder can sometimes go for years, giving the patients a " golden

window of opportunity " to improve and maintain their physical and mental wellbeing while their muscle memories are essentially intact with locomotive abilities.

Walking is the exercise you can enjoy and benefit from even at ripe old age without causing damage to the joints. There is a lot of mention about walking 10,000 steps a day as a magic number; realistically, walking 10,000 steps a day seems unattainable most of the people even with good intention. Research has shown that a daily walk around 7,500 steps regularly can give you very similar health benefits as 10,000 steps. Studies from Harvard University published in JAMA Internal Medicine recommends aiming for 4,400 to 4,500 steps per day to significantly cut mortality risk.

Walking as an exercise is a complex behavior and a very healthy bodily function, but many of us in our modern, digital world have taken it for granted, or simply forget about it; we become sedentary, night and day without realizing the serious consequences for our general health. The high cost of a sedentary lifestyle or physical inactivity just became more evident with a new global study showing that physical inactivity drive one in fourteen deaths. These findings, based on population data for 15 health outcomes across 168 countries, were published in March 2021 in the British Journal of Sports Medicine.

Many studies have linked sedentary lifestyle to the development of dementia. Regular physical activity helps reduce the risk of cognitive decline. According to some studies, researchers have reported up to a 50% reduction in the risk of dementia in older people who maintained regular physical activity. Data from the Aerobics Research Center in Dallas, Texas, found that physically active men lowered their risk of stroke by over 50%, and the risk reduction of stroke among physically active women was little better. Incidentally, people who don't perform regular physical activity are more likely to become depressed and/or gain weight; and both depression and obesity are modifiable factors to reduce the risk of dementia.

Going to the gym or going for a walk in the park you are not only exercising your muscles and your heart, but also your brain. Regular physical activity helps your brain form new neural connections, generates cell growth, and supplies your brain including its crucial areas with blood carrying oxygen and nutrients. A recent study of cognitively impaired, older adults, which was published in the Journal of Alzheimer's Disease found that taking brisk, 30-minute walks promotes healthy blood flow to the brain and improves performance while boosting memory function.

Many studies have shown the positive and beneficial impacts of exercise on the reduced risk of dementia. One notable study was published in the Journal of Applied Physiology in July 2021, with researchers at the University of Texas Southwestern Medical Center looking into the connection between Alzheimer's and other forms of dementia and exercise. The year-long study enrolled 70 men and women aged 55 to 80 with mild cognitive impairment (MCI), which tend to progress to Alzheimer's disease in 50% of the MCI cases. The participants were divided into two groups: one group was assigned to do brisk walking 25 to 40 minutes, 4 to 5 times a week. The other group took part in stretching class without aerobic component. The researchers found that the walking group saw increased motor skills, improved memory and cognitive function, in addition to improved cardio-fitness. The group assigned to do stretching and toning activities for a year did not show any appreciable improvements in cardiac and cognitive functions. The findings of this study revealed the importance of aerobic exercise for improving both cardiovascular and brain functions; the brain is a unique organ, requiring blood flow and oxygen-nutrient supply constantly.

More and newer research has added to the evidence that exercise can improve cognition, especially later in life. The study, conducted by scientists in the U.S., Canada, and Spain, found that older people who regularly exercised had greater levels of proteins crucial for brain health., compared to those who did not exercise. These differences were apparent even in people whose brains otherwise showed signs of dementia, suggesting that exercise could slow down the progression of cognitive decline and dementia. A lot of scientific data have suggested that prolonged, sedentary time could impair glucose and lipid metabolism, which were clearly recognized as risk factors for cognitive decline. There is a preponderance of the evidence that exercise may help safeguard the brain as you age; exercise increases the glucose metabolism of brain and decrease insulin resistance.

The act of walking requires functional integration of sensory and motor interactions; it activates the brain and the musculoskeletal system. One of the most important components of walking is balancing. In order to maintain the body's balance unconsciously and effortlessly as it changes position and moves over somewhat uneven terrain in a gravitational field, the brain needs and interacts with different information. It relies on a mechanism in the inner ears responsible for sensory orientation in three-dimensional space. If this function of inner ears fails, one cannot maintain equilibrium.

Besides the ears, the brain also requires visual input of information from other senses to keep the walking person in balance from tactile r3eceptors which let the brain know which part of the body is in contact with the ground, and from the proprioceptors in the muscles, tendons and joints that keep the brain continuously informed of the exact position of each part of the body in space. Dysfunction in any of these neural circuitries can lead to erratic movements and falling.

The cerebellum, located below the occipital lobes of the cerebrum, processes all of these sensory input to coordinate responses of muscles to the ever-changing requirements of ambulation. Research shows that exercise stimulates the sensory and motor cortex and maintains the brain's balance system. These functions begin to deteriorate gradually as we get older, making us prone to falling and becoming home-bound and bed-confined. Nothing accelerates the atrophy of the brain more than being immobilized in the same environment with little mental stimulation.

According to neuroscientific research, physical activity like walking stimulates the production and release of brain-derived neurotrophic factor (BDNF), a neuronal growth factor and a protective protein for the brain. This is found to improve learning and memory, according to many studies. In a 2011 meta-analysis of 15 studies that followed more than 33,000 people for up to 12 years, physical activities such as walking provided a buffer against cognitive decline and poor memory with its many other health benefits, both physically and mentally. BDNF plays a crucial role in effecting neuroplasticity and cognitive function, and the growth of new neurons.

Walking, like other forms of aerobic exercise, is a stimulator of ' mitochondrial biogenesis '; it increases the number and size of mitochondria in the muscles, allowing them to become more efficient at extracting oxygen from the blood. Research has shown that energy shortage in the brain due to dysfunctional mitochondria increases the risk for development of Alzheimer's dementia.

Walking, like other aerobic exercise or physical activities, can slow down the age-related changes of the brain, such as tissue losses in the cerebral cortex, hippocampus and the cerebral white matter. The amount of shrinkage or atrophy from the aging process, in unchecked, is most dramatic in the hippocampus, as much as 30% loss. Movement or physical activity is a natural function, and it should be maintained, if at all possible and as long as possible. The amount of exercise is thought to be at least 150 minutes a week, but any amount of physical activity can do the aging brain, as long as it can be done on a regular basis. Try to incorporate an exercise such as walking into your lifestyle, making it enjoyable and sustainable rather viewing it negatively like a chore.

If you live near nature, the woods, forest preserve or a park, you will reap additional benefits by walking in the natural surroundings with fresh air; the health benefits are measurable physically, mentally and psychologically. According to studies conducted in Drexel University's College of Nursing and Health Professions, the research team discovered that people who were more connected to nature tended to consume more fruits and vegetables than their more indoor-based peers. Their findings conclude that " Nature has been associated with better cognitive, psychological and physical health, and greater levels of environmental stewardship. "

Obesity --- Losing weight is not easy for most people, but losing weight and keeping it off is even harder. A Gallup survey published in February of 2016 showed that the obesity rate in the U.S. surged to a new high of over 32%, an almost 7 percent point increase since 2008. This means an increase of about eight million adults in the

U.S. who are dangerously overweight over a seven-year period, from 2008 to 2015.

Obesity is a chronic, treatable disease associated with excess weight and fat accumulation; it is a condition in which a person has an unhealthy amount and/or distribution of body fat. Currently, about 70% of the U.S. adults age 20 and older are overweight or obese. Lamentably, the percentage of children and adolescents who are overweight or obese has also increased. In 2011-2014, about 17% of U.S. youth ages 2 to 19 years old were obese; in 1988-1994, by contrast, only about 10% of 2 to 19-year old were obese. Obesity has indeed become an epidemic in many countries including the U.S., and an alarming global public health challenge.

To measure obesity, researchers commonly use a scale known as the body mass index (BMI). BMI is calculated by dividing a person's weight (in kilograms) by their height (in meters) squared (commonly expressed as kg/square meter. The normal range is from 18.5 to 24.9; overweight has a range from 25 to 29.9, and an obese person is between 30.0 to 39.9. Anything above 40 is considered severely or morbidly obese. It is beyond the scope of this book to look into the different diets, weight loss methods and treatments.

We have witnessed a double or triple escalation in the prevalence of obesity in the last two to three decades, probably due to urbanization, sedentary lifestyle, automation including automobiles, and increased consumption of high-calorie processed food. Obesity prevention is a critical factor in controlling diseases such as diabetes, cardiovascular disease, stroke, hypertension, some cancer and dementia. According to the Centers for Disease Control and Prevention (CDC), people who are overweight or obese, compared to those with healthy weight, are at increased risk for many serious diseases and health conditions. These include:

- High blood pressure
- Premature death from all causes
- Hyperlipidemia and dyslipidemia
- Type-2 diabetes
- Coronary artery disease

- Atherosclerosis
- Stroke
- Gall bladder disease
- Osteoarthritis
- Sleep apnea
- Some types of cancer
- Mental illness such as depression and anxiety
- Difficulty with physical functioning
- Lower quality of life
- Dementia

More and more studies have linked obesity to higher risk of developing dementia; ironically, obesity and dementia are two significant concerns in the modern world as both are increasing at an alarming rate. At UCL Institute of Epidemiology and Health Care, researchers found that people whose BMI was 30 or higher (at obese level) at the start of the study period had a31% greater risk of dementia at an average follow-up of 11 years, than those with BMIs at the normal levels. When BMI and waist circumference were considered in combination, obese study participants of either gender showed a 28% greater risk of dementia compared to those in the normal ranges. It is possible that the association between obesity and dementia might be potentially mediated by other conditions such as hypertension, diabetes, and cardiovascular disease, even though many studies have shown the independence of these confounding factors.

Researchers of University-College, London analyzed a large group of participants from the English Longitudinal Study of Aging (ELSA) who were at least 50 years old when enrolled in the study. Baseline measurements, including BMIs and waist circumferences, were collected at the beginning. They were followed up on an average of eleven years later to determine whether these participants had developed dementia.

Researchers found that participants who had BMIs corresponding with overweight or obese were more likely to develop dementia. They also noticed that abdominal obesity with high waist circumferences, a dementia risk, affected women more than men. Furthermore, the researchers stated that the linkage between obesity and dementia was independent of whether the participant was a smoker, had hypertension or diabetes, or carried the APOE4 gene, a genetic risk factor for Alzheimer's disease.

There are a few proposed mechanisms underlying the connection between obesity and the increased risk of cognitive impairment (dementia); these include dysfunctional adipocytes, insulin resistance, long-term inflammatory processes, imbalanced gut-brain axis, systemic bio-mediators, and decreased blood supply to the brain. One recent study published in the International Journal of Epidemiology, and supported by the National Institute on Aging, suggests that the accumulation of excess fat cells leads to damage to the white matter of the brain, and obesity may be associated with increased risk for developing dementia.

There is a big body of evidence that obesity is a modifiable risk factor for dementia; lifestyle changes such as regular exercise and proper diet are the mainstay of treatment. The discussion of weight is always a sensitive issue, sometimes it can get political; but, maintaining a healthy weight is about health, wellbeing and quality of life, and not merely about appearance. We must admit that obesity is a global health issue and problem, and its disease burden on society has not lessened.

Last but not least, a population-based study using BMIs and cancer incidence data from the GLOBOCAN project estimated that, in 2012 in the United States, about 28,000 new cases of cancer in men and 72,000 in women were attributable to overweight or obesity. A 2016 study summarizing worldwide estimates of the fractions of different cancers due to overweight/obesity reported that, compared with other nations, the United States had the highest fractions attributable to overweight/obesity for colorectal cancer, pancreatic cancer, and postmenopausal breast cancer.

Nevertheless, the longer a person stays fat, the more likely they are to develop bowel cancer, according to new research. This finding is based on a study of more than 10,000 participants who were tracked for almost two decades. Those with high BMIs and abdominal circumferences were two-and-a half times more prone to colorectal cancer than peers who maintained a normal body mass index. The medical scientists suggest that, as one of the mechanisms, the adipocytes from the excess fat release chemicals causing chronic inflammation – a cumulative toxic effect. This study published in the journal JAMA Oncology reveals unhealthy lifestyles are a much bigger factor than previously feared, augmenting the risks for development of various serious diseases including cancer, diabetes, cardiovascular and even dementia.

The association between greater adiposity and body fat and higher risk of cardiovascular disease have been well-established, obesity also increases the risk of cognitive decline. This is further supported by a study of older, overweight people in Dublin, which found an association between adiposity, particularly central adiposity, and reduced cognitive function. According to the researchers in the study, inflammation may play a major role in cognitive impairment in those who are overweight or obese. These obese individuals have high levels of plasma CRP, an inflammatory marker.

I call obesity "the evil master of health risks " because obesity causes multiple organ damages of the body, with its toxic, harmful and inflammatory abdominal or visceral fats. In 2008, data from a Permanente study of 7,000 volunteers, aged 40 to 45, showed that those with bellies (abdominal fat) are more likely to develop Alzheimer's disease later in life than those without abdominal fat. One theory postulates that the visceral fats send damaging molecules through the blood stream to the brain.

Air Pollution --- This is another modifiable risk factor to impact the development of dementia. According to researchers at the USC Keck School of Medicine, they studied more than 2,200 women between the ages of 74 to 92 and found that those who lived in areas with greater reductions in air pollution experienced fewer cognitive problems like memory loss. People living in and breathing cleaner air tended to have a slower decline in cognitive function, equivalent to 1 or 1.5 years. There are other studies that have linked air pollution to increased dementia risk.

On July 26, 2021, several studies were presented at the Alzheimer's Association International Conference 2021 in Denver, demonstrating that improving air quality may improve cognitive function and reduce dementia risk. Evidence of these studies at the AAIC-2021 also supported previous reports that have linked long-term air pollution with accumulation of Alzheimer's disease-related brain plaque, a possible biological connection. Among the key findings with the new data at AAIC-2021:

- Reduction of fine particulate matter (PM2.5) and traffic-related pollutants (NO2) per 10% of the Environmental Protection Agency's current standard over 10 years was associated with 14% and 26% reductions in dementia risk, and slower cognitive decline, in older U.S. women.
- Reductions of PM2.5 concentration over 10 years was associated with a reduced risk of all-cause dementia in French individuals by 15% and of Alzheimer's disease by 17% for every microgram of gaseous pollutant per cubic meter of air.

Undoubtedly, both the elevated levels of air pollution and the increasing number of dementia cases are becoming global public health crises. We are now seeing scientific data showing that improving air quality may actually reduce the risk of dementia; it is very important for federal and local governments, and businesses to adopt policies to reduce air pollutants, and to reinforce air quality standards to promote healthy aging.

There is an interesting study published in the journal Environment International, showing a relationship between levels of pollutants in the atmosphere and the risk of getting a stroke. According to the study, for every 10 micrograms per cubic meter of nitrogen dioxide in the air, the risk increases by four percent. When the amount of fine particulate matter, another pollutant, is increased by 5 cubic micrograms, the researchers saw the same percentage increase of dementia risk. Every extra cubic microgram of soot in the air raises the risk of a stroke by five percent. All these increases of dementia risk are spre4ad equally across the population, independent of age, smoking habits or socioeconomic factors. In contrast, they found that having an abundance of green spaces near your home may cut your risk of a stroke by up to 16 percent. As we know, stroke is a major contributing risk factor for dementia, and is found in at least 30% of Alzheimer's patients.

Air pollution remains to be a big and immediate environmental threat to human health, leading to millions of premature deaths every year and loss of millions of years of life. It has been linked to a variety of adverse health effects, including heart and lung diseases, cancer, neurological dysfunction, and birth outcomes. We all should participate in improving air quality and reducing air pollution as an individual in support of policies for a healthy environment because air pollution impacts all of us. According to the World Health Organization (WHO), majority of the world population are living in places where recommendations for air quality are not met. We must, at all times, remind ourselves to think broadly about how air quality and our environment can affect our health.

Low levels or Lack of Social Contact --- this is a sensitive and potentially dangerous personal and social issue, with significant impact on cognitive health. Social isolation or loneliness is entirely different from solitude, which is a voluntary and spiritual retreat as practiced by some religious groups or individuals like the Tibetan monks. According to the U.S. Government statistics, more and more older people in the U.S. are living alone, and the trend, unfortunately and woefully, will continue because the geriatric population is the fastest growing segment, not only in America, but also in the world.

Social isolation and Loneliness are interchangeable in the minds of most people, In actuality, they are two different states of mind and conditions. Social isolation is a state of complete or near complete lack of contact between an individual and society; it can be an issue for anyone at any age --- an unhealthy disconnection. Loneliness is usually temporary, and an involuntary lack of contact with other people. Of course, being alone is not the same as ' being lonely '; the desire by some people to feel peaceful, creative and restorative can be healthy and beneficial. Feeling lonely can be draining, distracting and upsetting; when this becomes chronic, it can lead to social isolation. One can feel lonely regardless of the levels of social contact. It is important to realize why you feel lonely, because only then you can see how you might address it.

One can feel lonely in a room full of people. There are two types of loneliness: ' state loneliness ' is something we have all experienced at times – being temporary and situational. But some people can suffer from ' chronic loneliness ', and that feeling never goes away. Social isolation and loneliness in older adults are serious public health risks affecting a considerable number of people in the United States and increasing their risk for dementia and other serious medical conditions, according to many social studies. A report from the National Academies of Sciences, Engineering, and Medicine (NASEM) points out that more than one third of adults aged 45 and older feel lonely, and nearly one-fourth of the elderly aged 65 and older are considered to be socially isolated. These older adults are at increased risk for loneliness and social isolation because they are more likely living alone, with loss of family and friends, and suffering from chronic illnesses. The situations for some of them, especially with impairments of hearing and vision can be much worse with potentially devastating health consequences.

Recent studies found that:

- Social isolation was associated with about a 50% increased risk of dementia,
- Social isolation significantly increased a person's risk of premature death from all causes, a risk that is similar to smoking, obesity, and physical inactivity.
- Social isolation and/or loneliness were associated with a 29% increased risk of heart disease and 32% increased risk of stroke.
- Both social isolation and chronic loneliness were linked to higher rates of depression, anxiety, and suicide.

- People who are socially isolated or feeling chronically lonely tend to have increased hospital admissions and emergency department visits.

Researchers retrospectively analyzed data from the population-based cohorts in the Framingham study, which was conducted over a 70-year span (1948 through 2018). Loneliness is this study was defined as the feeling of loneliness on three or more days a week. Out of the 2,308 participants, with average age of 73 and 56% women, none of them had dementia at the start of the study. 14% (329) developed dementia within 10 years. The calculations of the results indicate a 10-year dementia risk that is at least 50% higher for lonely adults, compared with not-lonely adults. According to further analyses of this research, loneliness is linked to poorer executive function, a lower overall cerebral volume, and greater damage to the white matter.

The states of social isolation and chronic loneliness are very unhealthy, both physically and mentally; it is a set-up for senility and frailty, and for everything that can go wrong with the body and mind. Human beings are highly social species, and we are meant to live in tribes, families and communities with inter-personal connections. When you are disconnected, you find no meaning or purpose in life. Without an enriched surroundings, with the absence or near absence of social interactions and sensory stimulations for the brain, there is no question that social isolation and loneliness serve as a strong risk factor for the development of dementia, especially Alzheimer's disease. Alzheimer's disease has grown considerably in proportion to the changing patterns of our modern-day society. The antidote to the withdrawal from life in this " disconnection syndrome " of Alzheimer's sufferers will not be found , wholly and solely, in the technologies of modern medical science despite three or more decades of intense search for a cure. We, humanity, must do some serious soul-searching with heightened social awareness and positive cultural changes in our battle against this horrible, dementing illness, and dementia in general.

People generally are social by nature, and quality social relationships can help them live longer, healthier lives. Our healthcare systems are an important, yet under-utilized partner in identifying loneliness and preventing medical conditions associated with loneliness. As we know, almost all adults aged 55 or older interact with the health care system in one way or another. For those without social connections, a doctor's appointment or visit from a home health nurse may be one of the few in-person encounters patients have. This truly represents a unique, timely opportunity to identify people at risk for loneliness pr social isolation!

Conclusively, maintaining social ties can not only reduce the risk of dementia, but also is linked to longevity. If you feel lonely or socially isolated, or have difficulty finding and making friends, get a pet. At the 2022 meeting of the American Academy of Neurology, data were presented to outline how sustained relationships with companion animals could keep your brain healthy. The health benefits of the human-animal bond were even stronger for long-term pet owners. The open and loving human-animal relationship involves cognitive engagement, social interactions, physical activity and having a sense of purpose and responsibility all contribute to the physical and mental well-being, reducing the risk for the development of dementia.

Traumatic Brain Injury (TBI)

--- Any violent blow or jolt to the head or body hard enough to cause injury to the brain, resulting in internal damage to the brain cells and increasing the risk for development of dementia, especially the insult to the head is repetitious. This is seen in certain contact sports such as boxing, American football, wrestling, hockey, and soccer even with younger players in good health. An object that goes through brain tissues, such as a bullet or shattered piece of the skull can also cause traumatic brain injury. In a study published in 2018 that included data on almost 2.8 million people in Denmark, collected over 36 years, researchers reported that traumatic brain injuries were associated with a higher risk of dementia, approximately 1 in 10 people who sustained a major traumatic injuries did develop dementias. It is estimated that 1.7 million Americans a year suffer traumatic brain injury resulting in changes in the brain structure and function, as well as thinking and memory difficulties, which can be either temporary or permanent. Of the 1.7 million cases of TBI, 275,000 required hospitalization and 52,000 died.

The symptoms of TBI are variable, depending on the extent and frequency of the injury; mild traumatic brain injury may affect your brain cells temporarily, while more serious TBI can result in long-term complications or death. Symptoms of TBI may appear immediately after the trauma, while others may appear days or weeks later. The symptoms include, but not limited to:

- Loss of consciousness for a few second or a few minutes
- Nausea or vomiting.
- Headache
- Fatigue
- Loss of balance or coordination
- Blurred or double vision
- Dizziness or vertigo
- Dilated pupils
- Convulsion

Mental or cognitive symptoms:

- Mood swings
- Alexia
- Depression
- Anxiety
- Coma
- Confusion
- Combativeness
- Slurred speech

TBI is a well-established risk factor for dementia. Studies have shown that neurodegeneration and progressive brain atrophy with cortical thinning occur after traumatic brain injury, including minor ones like concussion. TBI is a major problem in modern societies, primarily as a consequence of motor vehicle accidents and falls. So, you must protect your head at all times. It is important to wear seatbelts when riding as a passenger or driving behind the wheel. Seat belts, coupled with air-bags, do save lives and minimize any direct head trauma in case of an accident, or sudden, forceful stopping of the vehicle. If you enjoy bicycle-riding, wear your helmet. Besides the individuals participating in contact sports, other people at risk for TBI include children, especially newborns to children 3 to 4 years old. Older adults aged 60 and over are also prone to traumatic brain injury.

Alcohol Consumption

--- alcohol use is widespread in the United States, and it is readily available anywhere. According to a 2020 survey, about half of all Americans aged 12 and older were current alcohol drinkers. Admittedly, alcohol-induced dementia is a pressing, public health issue in our society nowadays.

Some studies have found that moderate drinking can be beneficial for health such as increasing lifespan, but many others suggest that the healthiest amount of alcohol consumption is none at all to avoid any potential medical and social problems. Multiple research and observational studies have demonstrated that people who drink high amounts of alcohol, more than three or more drinks a day, are at increased risk of developing dementia due to alcohol-related brain damage.

However, drinking alcohol in moderation has not been conclusively linked to an increased dementia risk, nor has it been shown to offer significant protection against developing dementia.

In the Whitehall Cohort Study in London, 9087 participants with a 23-year follow-up, the researchers came up with the following findings: the risk of dementia was increased in people who abstained from alcohol in midlife or who consumed high amounts of alcohol. The guideline is to encourage downward trend in consuming the amounts of alcohol to promote cognitive health.

We can see that alcohol and dementia are a complex relationship, from non-consumption, moderate consumption to heavy consumption with potential of alcohol use disorders. Imaging tests of the brains of heavy alcohol drinkers do reveal decreased neurons, brain atrophy with loss of white matter, similar to the changes in the brains of people with Alzheimer's disease. People with the APOE4 variants should abstain from any alcohol due to a higher chance of developing dementia, according to many studies.

Impaired vision --- Researchers at the University of Manchester, England, have found that, vision, like hearing, is also important for brain health. They studied 2,000 older adults the England Longitudinal Study of Aging after their successful cataract surgeries and found that improved vision slowed their cognitive decline by as much as 50%.

Evidence is undoubtedly emerging that undergoing cataract surgery can lower the risk of dementia by an average of 30%, according to a study published in JAMA Internal Medicine. The benefit lasted for at least 10 years and was specifically associated with a lower risk of Alzheimer's disease. Another study conducted by researchers at the University of Washington School of Medicine with more than 5,000 participants older than 65 from Kaiser Permanente Washington. They found that those who originally did not have dementia, after cataract surgeries, were 30% less likely to develop any form of dementia for at least 10 years after the surgeries.

Cataract is a condition affecting the eyes that causes clouding of the lens. Over time, a progression of the cataract eventually, if not treated, may result in vision loss. Cataracts are common in the elderly group, with more than three million cases a year in the U.S. This common eye problem is treatable by medical professionals, the ophthalmologists. It is unquestionable that dementia and vision impairment are interconnected, and research studying the linkage is on-going. Researchers hypothesize that it may have something to do with better quality sensory input traveling from the eyes to the brain after cataract surgery. Some special cells in the retina are associated with cognition and regulate sleep cycles, and these cells respond well to blue light. The lenticular opacities or cataracts block the blue light, and cataract surgeries could have reactivated those cells.

Vision loss in older people can occur due to eye conditions such as cataract, macular degeneration, or diabetes. However, people with dementia can experience changes in vision not related to the eye itself, because the dementia affects parts of the brain associated with visual input from the eyes. Each type of dementia can affect the visual system in the brain in a different way. The process of seeing involves many steps. The eyes send information to the brain, where it is interpreted in relation to expectations of what will be seen. The other senses, thinking and memories play a role as you become aware of what is being seen –the perception.

When you are unable to see very well, this will lead to reduced physical activity; you will be less likely to take part in hobbies, social events, and everyday activities such as reading, watching TV or a ball game. The social difficulties and withdrawal from life due to visual impairment in old age can certainly compromise brain health, raising the risk for dementia. Understandably, this could also increase the risk for depression and social isolation. There is no question that impaired vision due to, but not limited to cataract, is associated with an increased risk of dementia, and is also a modifiable factor.

Since there is no cure for dementia at this time, we should be focusing on the modifiable risk factors that can lower the risk for development of dementia, along with population-level efforts and public health policy to prevent dementia, and to focus on early detection for intervention.

Sleeping habit as a modifiable risk factor

In the foregoing segments of this book, we discussed about the importance of sleep for good health and longevity. Sleep distances are a known feature of dementia, making it difficult to determine whether poor sleep is a causal factor of dementia or a symptom thereof. According to Mayo Clinic experts, poor sleep may affect up to 25% of people with mild to moderate dementia and 50% of people of severe dementia.

According to a 2021 study by NIH's National Institute on Aging, published in the journal Nature Communications, researchers analyzed data from about 8,000 British citizens without the diagnosis of dementia beginning at age 50. Between 1985 and 2016, the participants were assessed on different health measurements, including how many hours they slept a night. To ensure the accuracy of this self-reporting, participants wore accelerometers to objectively calculate the sleep time. At the conclusion of the study, 521 participants had been diagnosed with dementia, at an average of 77. The data revealed that participants in their 50s and 60s who reported getting six hours of sleep or less were at significantly increased risk of developing dementia later in life, up to 30%.

Your brain needs adequate sleep to consolidate memories. While we cannot confirm categorically that insufficient sleep or poor sleeping habit actually increases your risk of developing dementia, there are plenty of reasons why a good night's sleep might be good for brain health.

As research for a cure for dementia continues, taking preventative measures and adopting healthy lifestyles to decrease the risk of developing dementia become crucial. It is important for us to be mindful of cognitive fitness, building a healthy brain to prevent dementia.

Researchers followed more than 350,000 under the age of 65 in the UK Biobank, a large biomedical database, trying to understand the multi-dimensional risk factors for dementia in general. The participants at the baseline assessments did not have a dementia diagnosis, and they were followed until early part of 2021 in England, Scotland and Wales. The results were published in JAMA Neurology at the end of the studies. They looked at socioeconomic status, education, psychiatric records, drug and alcohol use, environmental exposure to toxins, genetics and general health data. The following 15 risk factors seem to be significantly associated with developing dementia early:

- Lower formal education
- Lower socioeconomic status
- The presence of two apolipoprotein E4 allelle
- Complete abstinence from alcohol

- Alcohol use disorder
- Social isolation
- Vitamin D deficiency
- High levels of C-Reactive Protein
- Reduced hand grip strength
- Hearing impairment
- Orthostatic hypotension
- History of stroke(s)
- Diabetes
- Heart disease
- Depression

Memory and Dementia

The role of memory is very pervasive in our everyday life. There is no one specific part of the brain solely responsible for all memories, though there are certain regions of the brain related to specific memory subsystems. In other words, memory is not a single system that relies on one neuro-anatomical circuit, rather, memory consists of multiple systems that can function independently of one another. Nevertheless, the hippocampus is a very important memory region of the limbic system, the oldest area of the brain; it is critical for the ability to learn new information.

One of the symptoms associated with dementia is memory loss; in Alzheimer's disease, it seems to be the prominent symptom in the early stages. However, memory loss is NOT always a symptom of dementia, but it can be. Certain age-related memory loss does not cause a significant disruption in one's daily life. For example, one might occasionally forget a person's name, friend or relative, but recall it later on. One might misplace their glasses or cell phone sometimes. These incidents in memory are usually manageable and they don't usually affect one's ability to work, live independently or maintain a social life. But, when memory loss begins to disrupt your work, hobbies, social abilities, inter-personal and family relationships, it is time to stop the denial and seek professional

An entity called Mild Cognitive Impairment (MCI), as opposed to the ' normal ' age-related memory loss, it generally involves a notable decline in some thinking skill and memory. For many people with MCI, the condition eventually progresses to dementia due to Alzheimer's disease or other disorder causing dementia. The number one cause of memory loss is simply getting older; as we get older, changes occur in all parts of the body, including the brain.

Occasionally, some memory slippage is normal as you age, such as misplacing your car keys, forgetting a word, or name of a person, or being unable to find your wallet in the house. These memory lapses are minor problems which can happen to all of us as we get older. This essentially benign condition is called age-related memory loss or " benign senescent forgetfulness ", and should not be confused with Alzheimer's disease. Some ' senior moments ' are part of age-related memory loss, which is reversible with the right mental exercises.

Nowadays, with the hectic, multi-tasking environment in our modern society, there is much attention and talk about memory loss. The pharmaceutical industries are touting many supplements to help your memory, and the efficacies of these so-called memory and cognition boosters are anecdotal at best. Under normal circumstances, the secret of memory is attention, and the secret of attention is motivation. If your attention is not in the right place and not at the right moment, you will not remember it no matter how good your memory is. In fact, most of our memory complaints in our everyday life stem from the lack of attention: nothing is recorded in our brain in the first place, hence there is nothing to recall. Quite often, we see but do not look, we feel without being aware of it, and hear casually without listening. After all, by paying attention, you will ensure that all the circuitries in the brain are open and active. By associating the image and message, you will make a better recording and impression on your memory track.

Some memory problems are benign, reversible and treatable when the offending, contributing causes are identified and corrected. The following is a list of conditions that can cause poor or sub-optimal memory, and temporary memory disruption and/or impairment:

- Anemia
- Dehydration
- Infections
- B-12 deficiency
- Folate deficiency
- Hypothyroidism
- Hypoxia

- Depression
- Anxiety
- Sleep deprivation and sleep apnea
- Loneliness and social isolation
- Poly-pharmacy with prescribed medications
- Stroke of certain region of the brain
- Use and abuse of illicit drugs
- Unhealthy lifestyle such as alcohol abuse
- Exposure to neurotoxic elements
- Stresses, causing memory glitches
- Minor, benign head trauma

Memory is a very complex mental function, and declining memory is a stressful experience, to say the least. There are two major memory systems:

1. Explicit (or declarative) memory:

   This allows us to consciously remember people, places and objects. This memory system also enables us to remember telephone numbers and addresses. If someone does not know the name of the capital of the United States, you can tell them that it is Washington, D.C. Explicit memory works with the medial region of the temporal lobes of the brain.

2. Implicit (or non-declarative) memory:

   This is the system which the brain uses for motor and perceptual skills that people do automatically, such as driving a car, riding a bicycle, or swimming. As a contrast from the explicit memory system, which interacts with and relies on higher, cognitive regions such as the medial region of the temporal lobes, implicit memory system depends on regions of the brain that respond to stimuli such as the amygdala, the cerebellum and the basal ganglia.

In other words, implicit memory system is usually well-preserved in old age, even in the early stages of Alzheimer's disease because the dementing illness typically does not affect the amygdala, cerebellum and the basal ganglia. That explains why the persons with Alzheimer's disease who are unable to remember the names of loved ones or familiar places can still ride a bicycle, play the piano, read a book and swim.

It is heart-breaking and unfortunate that explicit memory for facts, events, people, etc., degrades early in the course of Alzheimer's disease. Thus, the affected persons are more likely to lose their more recent memories first, and the older ones are the last to go. This is the general pattern seen in Alzheimer's patients whose lives are gradually erased in reverse order --- first the ability to recognize or recall the names of their most recent friends and the grandchildren. Then, the memory of their own children disappears, and lastly, recollections of their spouses and siblings fade into the void!

It is undeniable that a person cannot learn when there is no memory. Learning and memory are the two most wonderful abilities of our mind. Learning is the process whereby we acquire new knowledge about the world and around us, and memory is the process whereby we retain the knowledge over time. Memory is the wonderful, remarkable and necessary " glue " that holds our psychic or mental life together. Without this amazing, unifying force, our consciousness will be degraded and broken into many, many fragments, and eventually disconnected.

Deficit in our memory is the result from loss of synapses where neurons communicate. Many studies have demonstrated that the brain can re-grow synapses even in the early stages of Alzheimer's disease if the affected individual remain mentally active with appropriate brain stimulations. According to the recent neuro-scientific research, regular mental stimulation and challenge in older people can form new dendrites to facilitate chemical signals from one neuron to another, strengthening and expanding the cognitive or brain reserve. The adult brains do make new neurons, called neurogenesis, which does occur in the hippocampus and hippocampal neurogenesis is enhanced by learning and environmental enrichment.

Very few dendrites, the receptive processes of neurons, are present at birth. During the first year of human life, there is an enormous increase in the number of dendrites, to the extent that each cortical neuron has enough dendrites to accommodate as many as 10,000 synapses with other neurons. This expansive, far-reaching pattern of synapses enables the human cortex to function as the high-level center for learning, memory and reasoning.

To maintain your brain health, to improve your memory, and to reduce your risk of developing dementia, you should include physical activity in your daily routine, socialize regularly, eat a healthy diet, have adequate sleep, manage your chronic conditions, reduce stresses, embrace lifelong learning, using the brain frequently and in new ways. The neuroplasticity of our brain will enable the neurons to continue to grow throughout life with mental activities.

When the electrical potentials pass repeatedly between two neurons, that particular synapse is active and strengthened. This is like walking in a wood; the more walking traffic on the path, the more the walking path becomes obvious and clear, and the more likely this particular path or trail will be used again. If the neuronal pathways or circuits in the brain are not being used, they will degrade and degenerate, just like the walking path in the woods getting fainter and fainter due to lack of usage by walkers or hikers.

We all have had things that we wanted to remember, but could not many a times. There are ways you can improve and strengthen memories and recall:

- Playing games such as card games, chess and scrabble because these are fun and wonderful stimuli for concentration and memorization skills.
- Saying it out loud or self-talking is what many smart people do. It is a form of rehearsal, making things more distinctive and memorable.
- Read and read again.
- Looking, not just seeing inattentively and haphazardly, strengthening your visual memory.
- Sleeping well to eliminate metabolic toxic wastes

- Stress reduction and management.
- Eating a balanced, healthy diet.
- Regular exercise including walking
- Meditation, which require consistent and persistent practice to be effective.
- If you can find a way to relate it to your life, it will help.
- Use mnemonic
- Draw it. A picture paints a thousand words. Our mind recalls images better than rows and rows of words.
- Do one thing at a time. Too much multi-tasking can affect your working memory and long-term memory.

Our identity is the sum of our memories. Alzheimer's disease or dementia is the worst thing that can happen to anyone who can think because it takes the ability away! Indeed, Alzheimer's disease and related dementias degrade and shatter the core of humanity.

Inflammation and dementia

Inflammation is our body's natural response of the immune system to injury. Unfortunately, aging is accompanied by an increase in chronic, low-grade inflammation, known as ' inflammaging '; Chronic inflammation can become a silent killer because it can increase the risk of many chronic diseases such as cardiovascular diseases, type-2 diabetes, cancer, rheumatoid arthritis, asthma, depression and dementia. There are different inflammatory markers in our body, and one of them is C-reactive protein (CRP), which serves to assess the risk for heart disease and stroke. An increase in the levels of Interleukin-6 and alpha tumor necrosis factor, inflammatory markers in the Central Nervous System, seem to play a role in the age-related loss of memory and cognitive function.

Inflammation of the brain, according to neuro-scientists, promotes the formation of plaques and tangles in Alzheimer's patients, resulting in subsequent death of neurons. The harmful effects of inflammation on the brain are so vicious, insidious and destructive that Canadian researchers have described Alzheimer's disease as "arthritis of the brain ". Studies have shown that the levels of inflammatory mediators produced by the activated microglia in Alzheimer's brains are elevated, as compared with those normal older individuals.

Inflammation as a risk factor for dementia is currently an area of intense medical interest. Many neuro-scientific studies have already linked chronic inflammation to cardiovascular diseases, type-2 diabetes and cancer. There is a plethora of scientific evidence that chronic inflammation in midlife could set up a cascade of chain reactions, over time, leading to damage of brain cells resulting in shrinkage and eventually dementia. In the last decade, many researchers have suggested that the presence of a sustained immune response in the brain might increase the risk of developing Alzheimer's disease, with inflammation as a central, pathophysiological mechanism.

In the 1990s, several large epidemiological and observational studies were published indicating that the anti-inflammatory treatments used in diseases such as rheumatoid arthritis, showed protective quality against developing Alzheimer's disease as much as a 50% reduction in the risk for developing Alzheimer's disease in patients who are on long-term non-steroidal anti-inflammatory drugs (NSAIDs). The involvement of a neuro-inflammatory pathway as one of the mechanisms in the development and progression of Alzheimer's disease has drawn much interest and attention in medical research nowadays.

The ties between inflammation and dementia are growing stronger as more and more studies are revealing. In fact, newly published research has concluded that chronic inflammation in midlife might be associated with brain atrophy decades later as older adults. A study of 1,050 people as part of the Honolulu-Asia Aging Study have found that inflammatory markers may reflect not only peripheral disease, but also cerebral disease mechanisms related to dementia, and these processes are measurable long before clinical symptoms become noticeable and apparent.

In " Neurology ", the medical journal of the American Academy of Neurology, a new research revealed that following a particular food regimen can reduce the danger or risk of dementia. Researchers have recently investigated the link between inflammatory diets and the risk of dementia in older population in Greece, following and surveying a total of 1,059 individuals over a course of three years. They found that those consuming highly inflammatory diets with a high Diet Inflammatory Index (DII) score were at least three times more likely to develop dementia than those consuming anti-inflammatory diets with a lower DII score, -1.76 and lower. The findings were published in the medical journal, Neurology, further supporting the link between inflammation and neurocognitive diseases like dementia.

An anti-inflammatory diet is rich in fruits, vegetables, beans along with tea and moderate amount of coffee. These foods are good sources of beneficial vitamins and minerals, which can protect the cells from damage and prevent inflammation in the body. It is undeniable that diet plays an important role in our overall health, including the heart health and brain health. There is a growing body of evidence that what you choose to eat can affect your risk for diseases, and in this case, the risk of dementia.

" Let thy food be thy medicine and medicine be thy food ", a profound and popular phrase by Hippocrates (460-377 BCE), often used to emphasize the importance of nutrition to prevent and/or cure diseases. It is encouraging that more and more Americans are beginning to recognize that the foods we eat every day can have a profound effect on our mental and physical health, longevity and well-being. The average 4-year medical school curriculum spends less than 1% of all lecture time on nutrition and diet. In fact, one study found that only 13 to 15% of internal medicine resident physicians reported feeling qualified to offer nutritional-therapeutic advice to their patients. Nevertheless, the rising interest in food as medicine, supported by evidence-based studies, is an exciting opportunity for all healthcare providers and a promising, holistic viable option for patients.

As people get older, it is all the more important to decrease the chronic, low-grade systemic inflammation in the body – fighting Inflammaging. Some foods are very inflammatory such as:

- Highly processed foods
- Sugar, including high fructose corn syrup
- Red meat
- Alcohol
- Unhealthy oil
- Regular soda and candies with artificial colors and flavors
- Refined carbohydrates such as white bread and pastries
- Fried foods

Some foods that are known for their anti-inflammatory properties include:

- Fatty fish
- Fruits

- Vegetables, preferably dark, leafy green
- Broccoli and cauliflower
- Beans and legumes
- Nuts and seeds
- Berries, especially blueberries
- Green tea with its epigallocatechin-3-gallate (EGCG)
- Coffee in moderation
- Olive oil
- Mushrooms, high in phenols and antioxidants

There are a few potent anti-inflammatory spices you should incorporate them into your meals, such as:

- Turmeric
- Cinnamon
- Black pepper
- Ginger
- Cayenne (Chili peppers)

Recently, researchers from the United States, Greece, and Ireland conducted a population-based study involving both men and women to investigate the adverse effects of inflammatory diets on cognitive health. Until now, there has been little research into the effects of an inflammatory diet on cognitive decline, including memory. At least, we are able to measure the inflammatory potentials of different diets to recommend dietary interventions for cognitive health, an important lifestyle factor one can modify to fight inflammation.

In general, following a Mediterranean and plant-based diet is best for protecting yourself against chronic inflammation and cognitive decline. The Mediterranean diet is not a fad; it is a lifestyle choice. This famous diet is plant-heavy with vegetables, fruits, wholegrains, fish and pulses. Olive oil with healthy fats is used almost exclusively, while lemons are common staples in the kitchen. Red wine is consumed and enjoyed in moderation.

Researchers at Rush's Alzheimer's Disease Center in Chicago created the MIND diet, short for Mediterranean-Dash Intervention for Neurodegenerative Disease (or Delay) with ten beneficial foods as follows:

- Berries, especially blueberries
- Beans
- Fatty fish
- Olive oil
- Poultry (non-fried)
- Nuts
- Vegetables (dark, green and leafy)
- Hard-boiled eggs, 4 to 5 times a week
- Whole grains
- Red wine (resveratrol)

Researchers from the Chicago Rush University Medical Center found that adding in foods like pizza, sweets and pastries with added sugar, processed meats, fried things like French fries, and soda (regular or diet) reversed the cognitive health benefits from the Mediterranean diet. If you take a closer look at the components of the Diet Inflammatory Index (DII), most of them are included in the Mediterranean diet. As for the pro-inflammatory components of the DII, they are present in the "Western diets " in the form of pastries and sweet, butter or margarine, fried snacks and foods, and red or processed meat.

There are a number of medical tests to detect inflammation, and four of the most common ones include Erythrocyte sedimentation rate (ESR), C-reactive protein (CRP), Ferritin, and Fibrinogen. Currently, testing for inflammation is not a part of routine medical care for all adults; chronic inflammation may be silent and may not cause specific symptoms. A better approach is to get routine medical care and check-up by your healthcare providers to identify and treat the conditions due to harmful chronic inflammation.

Diet is not the only weapon you have to fight the terrible, health-destroying inflammation; other positive lifestyle changes are also beneficial such as:

- Aerobic exercise, from mild to moderate

- Maintaining healthy weight to get rid of the abdominal fat
- Making quality sleep for 6 to 7 hours every night
- Quit cigarette smoking
- Moderate use of alcohol, preferably red wine
- Find your own ways to reduce chronic stress, such as meditation, because repeatedly triggered stress hormones contribute to chronic inflammation

With inflammaging, the immune system increases the production of the pro-inflammatory mediators, which can reach the Central Nervous System and decrease the levels of Brain-derived Neurotrophic Factor (BDNF), a beneficial protein that supports the growth and maintenance of neurons. The role of inflammation in neurocognitive diseases such as dementia has been well-established. Thereby, decreasing the levels of systemic inflammation in our body may reduce the risk of development or severity of chronic disease including dementia.

In a recent, large study published in Transitional Psychiatry, researchers collected data from 500,000 participants enrolled in the UK Biobank with participants between 45 and 75 years old. The volunteers agreed to follow-ups after 9 years, and anyone who had a diagnosis of dementia at the onset of the study were excluded, with 377,592 remaining for the study. After analyzing the participants' health nine years later, researchers found that tea drinkers were 16% less likely to develop dementia than non-tea drinkers. Those who drank three to four cups a day were at the lowest risk. The researchers believe that the high amounts of antioxidants in black and green tea reduce the levels of oxidative stress in the brain. Oxidative stress is due to an imbalance of free radicals and antioxidants in the body, resulting in neuroinflammation which plays a role in the development of dementia.

According to the United Nations, the worldwide population of those aged 60 and over will grow to 2.5 billion by 2050. The geriatric population is the fastest-growing segment, and we must be preemptive and proactive in our fight against Alzheimer's disease and other types of dementia. Otherwise, the disease burden will be unbearable for all of us and societies!

Dementia's impact on the caregivers:

Nothing is more difficult, more challenging and heart-breaking than taking care of loved one who is losing, or has lost their mind, speaking from my personal experience. Most of the patients with Alzheimer's disease and related dementia, at least 75% of them are receiving their care at home from their family, either the spouse, a close relative, or adult children, or close friend. Without the family caregivers, often called the invisible second patients, people with dementia would have very poor quality of life, and would likely require institutional care early on. Only a small number of them are placed in nursing homes, usually in their late stages of the dementing illness. Some of these facilities may have special care units, called memory or dementia care, with staff trained to care for dementia patients. Medical advances and innovation are helping people to live longer, but we are also seeing rising rates of dementia cases. Unfortunately, the lives we are prolonging seem to be less fulfilling in many cases, and unacceptable by some people. That is why it is important and sensible to match the longer lifespan with health span.

For most of us, if not all of us, the fear of mental disability is greater than the fear of physical disability due to its stupendous impact on life and health. Numerous studies report that caring for a person with dementia is more stressful and exhausting than caring for a person with a physical disability. The desire and drive to care for a loved one with dementia is unquestionably noble and good, but caregivers, usually unpaid family member, are at a high risk of stress, anxiety, suppressed immune system, and poor attention to their own health. A caregiver in a home setting is unequivocally subject to tremendous to pressure and stress sustained over a long period of time with demands and uncertainty. Caring and managing for your loved one with physical and mental disabilities, interjected by periodic, unpredictable medical emergencies or night-marish episodes, is extremely grueling, frustrating and sometimes frightening!

The current estimate of individuals affected with Alzheimer's disease and related dementia in the U.S. is about 5.5 million. By the year of 2050, the number of patients suffering from Alzheimer's is expected to reach 15 million; globally, this most common form of dementia will affect more than 130 million people, according to the estimate by the World Health Organization. In 2007 approximately 10 million Americans were caring for a person with Alzheimer's disease or another dementia with most of the caregivers were spouses, followed by adult children, mostly female. The number of caregivers needed will considerably rise due to the expected demands. Taking care of your loved one with dementia at home is a totally uncharted territory for many people.

Keep in mind that you will live with experience many unexpected incidents or surprising episodes when taking care of someone with a dementing illness, and to you, these incidents and episodes do not make any sense at all. Unfortunately, expressing your anger and other negative feelings and emotions to the ' sick ' person often will make the matter worse because the disease makes it impossible for the impaired individuals to respond to your anger in a rational manner.

As a care giver, do not assume any competence of your loved one who has Alzheimer's or other related dementia. For example, when you are relaxing by the pool with your mentally impaired individual, even if the person has always been a good swimmer, because the affected person may lose the judgment or ability to handle themselves in the water. This holds the same truth when you and the patient are near a lake, or river, or ocean front on the beach. Here is a fairly common but very dangerous situation: an impaired or confused person in a car may open the door and attempt to get out while the vehicle in moving. Thus, seat-belts must be properly used and all car doors must ne locked at all times. Having a preemptive strategy is of paramount importance to avoid any accident

Despite the resilience of human beings and the steadfast devotion of the caregiver, our psychological/physiological balance can be pushed over the edge beyond the limits to adapt and respond. The pressures of daily living and coping along with uncertainty can reach a point where the caregiver is constantly in a state of hyper-arousal. With frustration, suppressed anger, tension and irritability, come the eventual feelings of helplessness and hopelessness. The challenges for the caregivers can be overwhelming, to say the least. Many studies have shown that depression is common among caregivers of Alzheimer's patients, and this is by all means, not surprising. Once depression sets in, it will lead to hormonal changes and a compromised immune system, resulting in a " break-down ". The unfortunate break-down is essentially a state of psychological exhaustion with loss of enthusiasm, energy, and drive for life. In some cases, the deepening depression can reach a point of requiring hospitalization and medications for the caregivers.

Some studies have found that the wounds of Alzheimer's caregivers took longer time to heal than those of a control group due to dysfunctional and dysregulated immune system. Interestingly, many of them continued to show decreased compromised immune responses even years after their mentally-impaired loved ones passed away. Indeed, the sustained in caring for someone with Alzheimer's disease and related dementia can age the immune system of caregivers prematurely, making them vulnerable and susceptible to many different illnesses.

Researchers in social science have observed that, although it may be at times difficult to admit how they feel, Alzheimer's caregivers often experience over time anger or deep-seated resentment towards those they love and care for – I call it reactive ambiguity. In fact, the feelings of anger and frustration can conceal their pain and grief inside at a deeper level.

Taking care of someone suffering from a dementing disorder such as Alzheimer's disease is likened to watching a slow-motion picture, waiting for the tragedy to unfold. Most of the people who take care of a friend or family with Alzheimer's disease or a related dementia do it alone. Ideally and understandably, caring for a person with dementia should not be just one person's job; everyone involved with the patient should share tasks and responsibilities to avoid and minimize the risk of break-down or burn-out on the main caregiver.

Many caregivers, despite their devotion and willingness, may continue to feel frustrated and angry subconsciously that the persons they are taking care are no longer the persons they used to be. Such slow-burning resentment, a subconscious emotion, may not be easy to acknowledge or accept because it is clearly and ironically in conflict with the caregivers' sense of love, devotion and duty. This reactive ambiguity or deep emotional predicament is very likely to adversely impact the caregivers' health and well-being with potentially immense costs to our society.

If you are taking care of your aging and ailing parent, spouse, or close friend, or other family member afflicted with dementia, more specifically Alzheimer's, you most likely feel drained and stretched, both in time and energy, not including financial pressures and expenses associated with the care. It is a long, formidable and painful journey for both the caregiver and victim of the illness. The psychic toll is actually the heaviest and unfathomable. Being a caregiver for your loved one with Alzheimer's disease is and will be the most difficult and saddest thing ever done and encountered in your life. With so many roles you have to take on: you are the patient's ally, protector, social organizer, comforter, cook, driver, prompter, initiator, book-keeper, plus more with the ever-changing situations and conditions, including unpredictable medical emergencies.

Both the caregiver and the patient experience despair, frustration and loneliness in parallel. It is very important for the caregiver to reach out for help. You need to take care of yourself also, and here are some suggestions:

- Remember that you cannot do it all by yourself. Don't be afraid to ask family members and friends to help. Have a meeting with all the willing caregivers to come up with a workable schedule weekly or monthly. The care schedule may be changed sometimes if necessary with the primary caregiver coordinating.

- You must ensure that you have adequate sleep and rest, including occasional naps during the day. When you are rested with sufficient sleep at night, you will feel better and manage better.
- Eat a healthy, balanced diet
- Keep up with your favorite hobbies; if you do not have, try to find one you may enjoy
- Spend time with friends to have a cup of coffee or tea, and to have time away from the patient. This is not being selfish --- you are taking on a very challenging, physically and mentally exhausting job with multiple responsibilities and overlaid with many mixed emotions. This will lessen the tension and pressure with some diversion
- It is a normal emotion to grieve for the losses in your loved one suffering from Alzheimer's and related dementia, but allow yourself to dream new dreams
- Get exercise as often as you can; if you find it hard to fit it into your schedule, then take a walk with a friend in the neighborhood or in the park
- Sing your familiar and favorite songs or turn on your favorite music radio station. You can do it alone or with your loved one. Studies have revealed that singing improves mental and emotional well-being. Other studies with residents of nursing homes who sang together showed significant reduction in stress, anxiety and depression, compared with those residents who did not participate in singing
- Learn as much as possible about your loved one's illness, and try to focus on his or her remaining abilities. First and foremost is the safety of the compromised individual you are taking care of because their depth perception and ability to judge can be dangerous.
- Seek support and friendship from other caregivers because there is strength in knowing that you are not alone
- Eating with your family as often as possible. Research has shown consistently that health benefits of communal eating extend beyond merely eating in the company of

others. It provide an opportunity for communications and re-connection, in addition to improved digestion. In a 2015 study published in the journal Appetite, people, especially the older ones who eat alone tend to have a poor appetite with unhealthy eating habits, leading to poor nutrition.
- Seek counseling --- when your coping skills are overwhelmed and things seeming to drift out of control, counseling can be a great help to you and your helping family struggling with providing constant care to the patient. Most people seeking counseling are not 'sick' 'crazy', or neurotic, or 'mental'; they are normal people who sometimes have difficulty coping with real problems. Getting counseling is not a sign of weakness. With the heavy burden you carry in coping with and caring for the impaired person you love, you can use and garner all the help you can get, and this is not a reflection on your strength.
- Praying for spiritual inspiration and support to find equanimity and peace. If you have a religious affiliation, find time to join your organization regularly. The positive impact of faith in the lives of 80% of the world's population who are involved in organized religion is undeniable. Many studies have shown that faith gives you a sense of meaning and purpose that can help overcome incredible adversity.

Sometimes, a wife with Alzheimer's disease will insist that you are not her husband. This can be very heart-breaking and emotionally unbearable. All you can do is to reassure your impaired spouse, "I am your husband", and avoid arguing. You also need to reassure yourself that it is not a rejection of you, because it is just an inexplicable confusion pf your spouse's brain. Occasionally, a caregiver may feel that the impaired patient is "seeing the dead". This phenomenon is called dementia-related psychosis, and this symptom is not uncommon during the advanced or final stages of dementia.

The negative aspects of caregiving for people with dementia tend to receive most attention, and it is rightly so; but caring for someone you love is also associated with positive feelings and outcomes. Social studies have revealed that, over half of the caregivers, have positive experiences such as enjoying togetherness, sharing activities, feeling a reciprocal bond, spiritual fulfillment and growth, stronger faith, and feelings of accomplishments. Currently, majority of people with dementia live developing countries, at least 60%. One of the main differences between caregiving in the developed and developing countries is the living arrangements, whereby individuals with dementia in the developing countries live in much larger households with extended families. This communal type of arrangements, personally speaking, seem to offer some cultural advantages from the perspectives of Alzheimer's disease and other dementia. As people, including caregivers and the patients, are living in large households, care is distributed among a greater number of family members with less strain, stress and pressure for the main caregivers.

It is unquestionable and undeniable that, with the chronic and constant stress and the intensive demands of their role, many family caregivers of loved ones with dementia suffer from depression and anxiety. Group therapy conventionally seems to have inconsistent results in reducing levels of depression in the caregivers. A special treatment modality, called Mentalizing Imagery Therapy (MIT), which is originally conceptualized by Felipe, Jain and Peter Fonagy, has been shown by researchers from the Massachusetts General Hospital at Harvard Medical School to be rather effective in relieving depression and anxiety and improving the well-being of caregivers.

Epilogue

While nobody is guaranteed a long life, there are some actions you can take to increase your odds. The foods that you eat everyday play an important and critical role, with some foods lengthening your life expectancy and others potentially taking a toll. Centenarians make up about 0.004% of the current world population, and these lucky few are not easy to categorize.

According to a large meta-analysis of scientific studies in the American Journal of Clinical Nutrition, eating pulses (chickpeas, beans and lentils) is associated with a lower death rate The risk of all-cause mortality decreased by 16% when intake of pulses increased to 150 grams (5oz) a day. Another study, funded by the Bill and Melinda Gates Foundation suggested that 82 million deaths globally could be attributed to a low intake of fruits. The risk of all-cause mortality decreased by approximately 10% when fruit consumption increased to 250 grams (8-9 oz) a day. According to the United States Dietary Guidelines, 9 out of 10 Americans do not eat the recommended amounts of vegetables, while 8 out of 10 Americans fall short on fruits. For good health and longevity, you must increase your intake of fruits and vegetables, and in so doing, you will leave less space on your plate for foods such as added sugars, artificial sweeteners, harmful chemical additives, red meat and highly processed foods.

Another study, also funded by the Bill and Melinda Gates Foundation, has suggested that excess salt intake was responsible for three million deaths globally in 2017. The UK's Action on Salt campaign states that high salt consumption causes high blood pressure, leading to strokes, heart disease and heart failure.

The American Institute of Cancer Research reports that all berries contain a range of anti-cancer compounds, but blueberries are particularly rich in anthocyanosides, which are potent anti-oxidants and anti-inflammatory. Blueberries have also been shown to improve brain functions. The flavonoids in blueberries have both antioxidant and anti-inflammatory properties.

According to the study by researchers of Norway's University of Bergen, published in PLOS Medicine: Changing from the typical Western diet to an " optimized diet " at age 20 could expect a lifespan increase of 10.7 years for women and 13 years for men. Even the change at age 60 can still add 8 more years of life for women and 8.8 years for men. At age 80, the gains are about 3.4 years for both men and women.

A Mediterranean diet has been regarded as the most acceptable and best diet for health and wellbeing consistently five years in a row, according to U.S. News and World Report. Furthermore, there is a plethora of evidence that Mediterranean diet may reduce risk of developing dementia. A large MRI brain trial related to diet over a period of 18 months was conducted recently by Israeli researchers at Ben-Gurion University of the Negev, collaborating with experts from Leipzig University and Harvard University. The 284 participants between the ages of 31 and 82 underwent MRI brain scans before and after the trial.

Specifically, the researchers measured hippocampal-occupancy (HOC) and lateral-ventricle- volume (LVV) as indicators of brain atrophy and predictors of future dementia. The researchers were surprised to see dramatic changes in 18 months identified by anatomical structures in the brain. The findings suggest that Mediterranean diet is protective of brain health, attenuating or slowing age-related cerebral atrophy. This is certainly a simple, safe and promising option for slowing or stalling age-related neurodegeneration of the brain by adhering to the Mediterranean diet, which may keep your brain young.

The Mediterranean diet is indeed an " optimal " diet for longevity. According to a study published in the journal PLOS Medicine, if a woman began eating optimally at age 20, she could increase her lifespan by over 10 years; for a man on the same " optimal " diet from age 20, he could add 13 years to his life. The study also stated that, by starting the healthy optimal diet at 60, a woman could increase her lifespan by eight years, while a man could add up to nine years to his life. The plant-based diet could even benefit 80-year-olds men and women who could add 3.5 years to their lifespan.

While it might be difficult to change your diet entirely, but you can add and include some of the beneficial elements into your diet slowly so that you can live a long and healthy life.

With a closer look at the people from the " Five Blue Zones ", homes to the largest concentrations of centenarians, one common physical feature is the absence of abdominal fat which is a strong risk factor for many health problems. Abdominal obesity is common in the United States, and I think it is one of the reasons for the decrease in life expectancy among Americans in the recent years. Learning from their simple daily habits and practices for longevity without abdominal adiposity, residents of the Blue Zone:

- Drinking plenty of water, not sugary beverages or diet soda
- Eating plenty of whole grains – many studies have concluded that there is a link between higher fiber consumption and lower risk of abdominal obesity, besides other health benefits from a high intake of fiber in the diet
- Consistent adequate sleep
- Regular physical activities, incorporating natural movements
- Eating smaller portions and following the 80% rule.
- A wise saying : " eat breakfast like a king, lunch like a prince, and dinner like a pauper. " Many studies have validated the importance of a healthy breakfast in the morning, and the negative impact of skipping breakfast. According to a study published in the Japanese Journal of Human Sciences, skipping breakfast as a daily habit can increase your risk of dementia by four times!

Over the years, I have visited quite a few nursing homes where my older family members, relatives and close friends received geriatric care in their last exit of the life journey. I am always amazed at their food trays during meal times because they lack most of the elements of the Mediterranean diet. Personally, I think the older residents at nursing homes, whether they are institutionalized for general supportive care and maintenance or for memory and dementia care, will feel better with improved mentation if there is more focus on the MIND diet. MIND stands for the Mediterranean-DASH Intervention for Neurodegenerative Delay or Disease. It combines components from both the Mediterranean diet and DASH diet (Dietary Approach to Stop Hypertension).

The components of the MIND diet are common and rather inexpensive, and some of them include vegetables, fruits, berries, olive oil, whole grains fish, beans and nuts. The choices of healthy vegetables are many and the list is long, and the following is just a guide to create healthy meals:

- Carrots
- Broccoli
- Asparagus
- Tomatoes
- Egg-plants
- Sweet potatoes
- Spinach
- Cauliflowers
- Brussels sprouts
- Beets

They are filled with immune-boosting antioxidants, fiber, B-vitamins and minerals. Many, many studies have linked multiple health benefits of increased intake of vegetables to decreased risk of chronic diseases, including cardiovascular disease, typy-2 diabetes, certain cancer, and neurodegenerative disorders like Alzheimer's and related dementias. Many researchers theorize that the MIND diet decrease DNA errors and somatic mutations due to reduced levels of oxidative stress. The evidence is more than suggestive, it is compelling!

The following is my favorite list of superfoods for the brain, and incorporating them into your healthy diet will help nourish your brain to stay sharp:

- Blueberries, including other berries
- Green tea
- Oily fish
- Walnuts
- Dark chocolate with at least 60% cacao or cocoa
- Eggs, preferably hard-boiled
- Dark leafy greens
- Pumpkin seeds
- Avocado
- Whole grains

According to a recent poll, most of the aging Americans want to stay in their homes and live independently for as long as possible – aging in place. Almost half of them with the survey and polling have little or no idea the steps needed for them to take in order for them to remain safely and comfortably at home in their old age. To make the situation for aging worse, many of the older Americans live alone, up to 25% of them. For these older American loners, they must have advanced planning for social support and assistance, in addition to safety and accessibility features of their homes. Some of these features include but not limited to:

- Ground-floor bathroom
- Door frames wide enough for a wheelchair
- Lever-style door handles
- Entrances with ramps or no steps
- Grab bars I, both installed in the bathroom, both the shower, tub and toilet
- Avoid area rugs which are fall risk
- Walker near bed for a trip to the bathroom due to nocturia
- Stay away from slippery flooring materials
- Easy access to emergency call button

A special note for people over 65 who have to wake up to pee at night:

Waking up at night to go to the bathroom seems like a benign annoyance, but it is a health risk because it increases your risk of falling with some severe health consequences. Nocturia can be caused by a number of factors such as drinking a lot of fluids before bedtime, diuretic medications, diabetes, or heart failure. With age, your bladder can weaken or lose elasticity and the ability to hold as much urine. Nevertheless, it is advisable to consult your physician if you have nocturia.

Our desire to live independently into old age is commendable, but an aging America needs to make some significant changes including the foods we are eating and the lifestyle we choose every day. In a society where youth is often valued over old age, shame about age becomes something that many of us carry around as we grow older. Didn't we use to respect aging and elderly people? Most instances of ageism are invisible and it is ingrained in our daily lives and our thinking. It is time for us to take off the blinders in order to see it clearly and make proactive changes.

It is unquestionable that healthy lifestyle choices have a positive, significant impact on our overall well-being. There is a plethora of evidence that if everyone were to pay attention and mindful of living a healthy, proactive lifestyle, the incidence of age-related illnesses after age 60 would dramatically decrease. It is never too late to change and start a healthy lifestyle!

As far as Alzheimer's disease and other related dementia are concerned, we are currently experiencing just the tip of the iceberg right now. According to the Alzheimer's Association, the cost of taking care of Alzheimer's and dementia patients in the U.S. will increase from $318 billion currently to $1 trillion by 2050 as the population ages. By identifying the factors that may raise dementia risk, we hope that a substantial portion of dementia cases can be prevented through public health interventions.

With the modifiable risk factors identified, theoretically dementias could be delayed or prevented. You can do something about those modifiable risk factors, and have nothing to lose but everything to gain. Dementia does not have to be part of your aging, and it is not pre-ordained and can be modified and altered.

It should be emphasized that individuals living with dementia are not just people who have been measured against a list of symptoms to meet the criteria of a specific diagnosis. Two older adults who are the same age, and have the same diagnosis and at the same stage of their cognitive decline, may have different signs and manifestation of dementia in their own different ways. The clinicians and supporting staff must look at the life experiences patients have had and their personality. The approach to dementia care should be person-centered care, focusing on individual personal experience as the basis and understanding their needs which include comfort, inclusion, attachment and identity with love at the center in order for them to thrive as a human being. Each case of dementia thus develops differently with somewhat different outcomes. In other words, people living with dementia are not all the same. We must not stigmatize them and accept each person for who they are.

Besides eating your way out of a potential dementia diagnosis, you can also ward off dementia by regular walking and exercise. Get moving. Sitting is the new smoking. The bonus is " walking your way out of dementia ". Our bodies are made for movements and physical activities. Human movement is a natural function, and it should be maintained as long as possible. I just can't emphasize enough the importance of exercise such as walking for your physical and mental health, and the older generation needs it even more.

Walking is a great form of cardio and aerobic exercise with numerous health benefits. Walking can increase the production and release of brain derived neurotrophic factor (BDNF), a protective protein in the brain to improve learning and memory due to synaptic integrity. In a 2011 meta-analysis of 15 studies that followed more than 33,000 people for up to 12 years, regular physical activity like walking provided a buffer against cognitive decline and poor memory, along with its many other health benefits, both physically and mentally.

Aerobic exercise including walking can slow down age-related changes of the brain, i.e. decreasing tissue losses in the cerebral cortex, hippocampus, and the cerebral white matter, with increased blood flow carrying oxygen and nutrients to the brain. The amount of shrinkage from the aging process, if unchecked, is most dramatic in the hippocampus, as much as 30% according to neuroscientific research. The neuro-protective benefits of regular exercise for just 20 minutes a day, 150 minutes a week, can still be viable in later phases of life. Thus, incorporating regular physical activity into your everyday life---no matter how young or old you are, is important and necessary for healthy longevity without dementia!

Just a few words about ' forest bathing ', taking a walk through nature: you will notice the sounds and smells around you with the birds chirping, a stream flowing nearby, falling leaves, small animals running up and down the branches of trees, and your feeling of the breeze. The experience of these micro moments of life during the walk in nature will bestow upon you with profound and massive health benefits, the mind in particular.

Researchers found that those who exercised frequently and regularly later in life were significantly less likely to have developed Alzheimer's disease and other forms of dementia by their time of death. A 2022 study published in the journal Alzheimer's and Dementia, states that later life physical activity is one of the most consistently recommended lifestyle modifications to support and enhance brain health and forestall cognitive aging. According to the recent report by the Alzheimer's Association, inactivity alone is estimated to account for up to four million dementia cases---a staggering significant number!

A study by the Cleveland Clinic published in the journal Neurology in 2021 revealed that those who performed frequent, regular physical activity scored better on memory and cognitive tests. " Every increase in physical activity by one standard deviation was associated with a 31% lower risk of dementia ", reported the Cleveland Clinic.

Delaying the onset of dementia or slowing the progression of dementia even for five years would have a massive social and economic benefit!

Health disparities in Dementia Care:

In the U.S., a big melting pot, Alzheimer's disease and related dementias are conditions with profound disparities, disproportionately affecting many racial and ethnic groups. The disparities in healthcare are especially significant for vulnerable populations such as the chronically ill and disabled, low-income individuals, rural communities, the LBGTQ population, and geriatric segment of our society. Health disparity refers to a higher burden of illness, injury, disability, or mortality experienced by one group relative to another. The term " health inequality " and " health inequity " are also used interchangeably with health disparity. In fact, health and healthcare disparities are not new, and they have been documented and recognized for decades. However, many barriers still exist in our current American health care system. Health disparity is closely linked with social, economic, and/or environmental disadvantage. People who are adversely affected with obstacles to health are often excluded and discriminated, based on their race and ethnicity, socioeconomic status, religion, physical disability, gender, sexual orientation, or mental health.

Stigma, misunderstanding, cultural differences and weak linkages to our nation's healthcare system has led to significant disparities in Alzheimer's and dementia diagnosis rates and access to care and treatments. As a case in point, whites make up the majority of the 5.5 to 6 million people in the United States with Alzheimer's disease. But, the evidence from many studies shows that African Americans and Hispanics are at higher risk for Alzheimer's and related dementias.

According to statistics from the Alzheimer's Association:

- African Americans are about two times more likely than white Americans to have Alzheimer's and other dementias.
- Hispanics are about one and one-half times more likely than whites to have Alzheimer's and other dementias.

Despite their higher rates due to higher risk than white Americans, African Americans and Hispanics are less likely than whites to have a diagnosis of the condition.

Furthermore, when they are eventually diagnosed, African Americans and Hispanics are typically diagnosed in the later stages of the disease. And at the time of their confirmed diagnosis, they are more cognitively and physically impaired, therefore, in need of more medical care with heavier and more costly social burden.

Unfortunately, the minority caregivers for their loved ones also face discrimination. Many surveys show that among non-white caregivers, more than half of them have experienced discrimination when navigating the health care system for their care recipients/patients. One of their main concerns is that healthcare providers or staff do not listen to or doubt what they are saying because of their race, color, or ethnicity. There could be some implicit bias, while cultural and language can also hinder patient-provider relationships.

The lack of consistent access to health care can have a negative impact on the person's physical and mental health. Access is undoubtedly important to give anyone the opportunity for regular preventive health services and early diagnosis of many medical conditions, such as diabetes, heart disease, hypertension, and dementia. Consistent, available access can help prevent hospitalization through effective management of chronic health conditions and coordination of care with family of the patients.

According to reliable estimates, the number of adults living with Alzheimer's disease and other forms of dementia will more than double over the next twenty years. It is a sad fact that more than 40% of dementia cases go undiagnosed nowadays. Early detection, diagnosis, and treatment of dementia are critical to protect individuals against risks from delay or missed diagnosis, and allow patients, their families and caregivers to plan for the future as the conditions progress.

The strain on the current American healthcare infrastructure will exacerbate as our aging population continues to increase. In fact, Alzheimer's disease has already become one of the leading causes of death in the U.S. The United Nations projects that by the year 2050, nearly two billion people the world will be over the age of 60. As a humanity, we must act now to hold back the tide of dementia!

As health care professionals, we have a responsibility to be aware of and to address our own biases, and how they show up in our practices in order to provide equitable, just and honest care for our patients and their loved ones.

Dr. Richard Ng, B.S., D.O.

Neurocognitive impact of long COVID

At the time of this writing, the number of coronavirus cases has reached about 521,000,000 (Five Hundred Twenty-One millions) with over six million deaths. The United States leads the number of cases at 84,200,000 (Eighty-Four million and two Hundred Thousand) approximately.

Our thinking that COVID-19 is more of a respiratory disease is actually not true; once it infects the brain, it can affect anything because the brain is the important central processor for everything. An international study from Lancet of people with long COVID documented over 200 different symptoms across 10 body systems. Most of the 3,762 participants in the study reported memory problems and cognitive dysfunction as the most persistent and pervasive symptoms. Brain fog is the most common symptom described by people with cognitive dysfunction following COVID-19 infection. In fact, neurologic complications from COVID-19 are common and can range from decreased mental clarity, the so-called brain fog, to stroke.

The neurological or cognitive symptoms of long COVID can occur months after the infection, and they can be debilitating for many people. Some affected patients may have problems concentrating, keeping up with conversations and multitasking. Some may lose their train of thought easily and have difficulty with memory. Other symptoms of post-COVID condition include fatigue, headaches, shortness of breath and trouble sleeping. The Centers for Disease Control and Prevention (CDC) define long COVID as " returning or ongoing health problems " occurring 4 weeks or more after contracting SARS-CoV-2, the virus that causes COVID-19.

A significant study was published online March 8, 2022 in JAMA Neurology, involving 1,438 COVID-19 survivors discharged from three COVID-designated hospitals in Wuhan. Before the participant/patients were infected, none of them had cognitive impairment. At 12-months post-discharge, 12.5% of COVID survivors had developed cognitive impairment. At 6-months post-discharge, 10% of those with severe COVID-19 had dementia, and at 12-months,

15% had dementia. The incidence of dementia and mild cognitive impairment was significantly higher in those severe COVID-19 cases than in the mild cases and controls.

A team of researchers reviewed 24 studies from 4 continents, covering more than 200,000 participants, measuring loneliness before and during the COVID-19 pandemic. They found that loneliness has increased markedly across the world during the corona pandemic by at least 5%. This should come as no surprise with the lock-downs, quarantines, social distancing, and closings (temporary or permanent) of places where people could socialize and promote bonding.

Many researchers identified COVID-associated brain damage months after the infection and were surprised by the reduction in the grey matter of the brain, representing up to 10 years of aging. The reduction of grey matter seemed to be more pronounced in the orbitofrontal and para-hippocampal gyrus, regions of the brain associated with smell. There is no question that cognitive decline post-COVID-19 including brain fog and mild cognitive impairment will boost global dementia rates, and this would significantly exacerbate the global burden of dementia and other neurodegenerative conditions in the post-COVID-19 era. The notorious post-COVID brain fog, characterized by loss of mental clarity and inability to concentrate, has thrusted this medical umbrella term into the spotlight with in creased interest and awareness.

Brain fog is definitely on the rise with millions of people reporting it worldwide. There are multiple causes of this medical condition, and its various symptoms include poor concentration, feelings of confusion, inability to focus, , slow thinking, fuzzy thoughts, forgetfulness, sometimes problem with language and finding worlds. According to recent research published, there may be distinct parallels between the impaired cognitive functioning of long-Covid and the dearly stages of neurodegenerative diseases such as Alzheimer's.

In closing, for longevity, the followings are non-negotiable:

- Sleeping 7 to 8 hours a night as a consistent habit
- Get moving, including daily walk
- Eat less, the 80% rule; eat early to avoid late night meal
- Drink more water
- Drink green tea, and coffee without sugar and cream
- Avoid processed foods
- Eat more plants and healthy fats
- Consume less meats (red or poultry)
- Get regular medical checkups
- Let food be thy medicine
- Stay socially connected with friends and families
- Find and pursue purpose and meaning in your life
- Work-life balance

In addition, the followings are important components of a brain protective lifestyle:

- Regular exercise
- Mental or brain stimulation
- Stay socially connected to prevent loneliness and isolation
- Get 7 to 8 hours of quality sleep every night
- Find own ways to relieve stress
- Follow a MIND or Mediterranean diets
- Protect your head
- Learn something new
- Control chronic health conditions, such as diabetes and hypertension
- Check your hearing and vision to ensure proper sensory input to the brain
- Stay away from cigarette, including second-hand smoke

Of course, a balanced diet that promotes longevity is also good for brain health, nevertheless, there are six nutrients, according to multiple studies, that can help ward off dementia or slow and delay its development:

- Magnesium – there is so much attention to this nutrient lately, and this is not surprising because Magnesium is involved in over 300 biologic and chemical reactions within our bodies. A 2023 study of men and women 40 to 73 years old found that more magnesium was linked to a greater brain volume. Brain cell loss is a natural part of aging, resulting in cerebral atrophy. Magnesium deficiency has been associated with neurodegenerative diseases such as Alzheimer's and Parkinson's.

    The recommended daily allowance for women 320 milligrams and 420 milligrams for men. It is preferable to get your magnesium in your diet, and good sources for magnesium include pumpkin seeds, spinach, almonds, peanut butter yogurt and black beans.

- Choline – an important component of cell membranes, most notably neurons. Choline serves as the raw material for acetylcholine, a neurotransmitter. It is one of the neuroprotectors to ward off brain cell damage. The body naturally makes small amounts of this nutrient, but it is not enough to fulfill your needs, so you need to get some from your diet.

    Foods that are good sources of choline include whole eggs with its almost entirely concentrated in the yolk. Organ meats like liver and kidneys are some of the best sources of choline Caviar or fish roe is an excellent source of choline. Seafood, including fish like salmon, tuna and cod. Shiitake mushrooms, soybeans, beef, chicken and turkey, almonds, cruciferous vegetables. Kidney beans and quinoa. Choline is easily available because you can get it from both animal- and plant-based foods.

- Omega-3 fats – according to American Heart Association, omega-e fats defend against cell destruction and protect arteries that nourish the brain. Not all omega-3 fats are created equal. Docosahexaenoic acid (DHA) and eicosapentaenoic acid (EPA) are associated brain health. Normal brain cells are particularly rich in DHA. Researchers have observed that higher levels of DHA in the blood delayed the onset of Alzheimer's disease by at least five years in people aged 65 and older without dementia. If you avoid fish for any reasons or only eat small amounts of fish, you may benefit from a supplement with EPA and DHA.
- Vitamin B12 – this nutrient helps maintain myelin, which coats some parts of neurons and ensures swift and accurate communication. Thus, it is required for the function of the Central Nervous System. It is required for healthy red blood cell formation, and DNA synthesis. Vitamin B12 deficiency is a known cause of cognitive decline. In fact, it is important to rule out B12 deficiency in anyone with cognitive decline and changes as it may be reversable.

People with inadequate vitamin B12 intake or regularly taking certain medications for gastric reflux disease or diabetes are at a greater risk for low vitamin B12 levels. Aging also reduces the body's ability to absorb natural vitamin B12 because older people produce less gastric acid required to process it. Vitamin B12 is found naturally only in animal foods or in foods of animal origin, including fish, meat, poultry, eggs, and dairy products.

- Proteins – the body uses the amino acids in food proteins to produce brain cells, neurotransmitters and other compounds that support brain health. One study followed 77,000 men and women for over 20 years and found that more protein was associated with less cognitive decline later in life. Protein requirements increase with age, especially

older people with a small appetite. Regularly consuming complete proteins – foods with all of the amino acids our body can't make is a good strategy for brain health.
- Fiber – this nutrient not only keeps the gut moving, but also keeps the brain healthy. Most people are familiar with the digestive health benefits of fiber, including weight control and its effect on cholesterol; a research was conducted with more than 3,700 men and women 40 to 64 years old who were followed for 20 years. They found that higher levels of fiber, particular the soluble kind were associated with less dementia.

Fiber is found naturally in plant foods. Many plant foods contain both soluble and insoluble dietary fibers, and the recommended daily intake of fiber for women is 30 grams, and 35 to 40 grams for men.

Like any part of the body, the brain needs love and attention, especially for older people. Actively involving the brain through healthy life style habits and proper nutrition can help boost memory and concentration as well as reduce the risk of neurodegenerative diseases like Alzheimer's disease.

As of this writing, there is still no cure for dementia despite all the efforts in the past few decades. However, we have learned a lot more about this syndrome and the diseases that cause it. With its multiple dimensionality and causality, the cure is not simple to be found in a bottle of pills or injections. Early detection seems to be the key to tackle it and to allay the anxiety and fear of the sufferer and his or her loved ones and caregivers.

www.ingramcontent.com/pod-product-compliance
Lightning Source LLC
LaVergne TN
LVHW021714060526
838200LV00050B/2652